5-Minute Balance Exercises for Seniors

How To Improve Stability, Posture, Mobility & Avoid Falls in Only 5 Minutes a Day with a 28-Day Home Workout Plan (50+ Easy-to-Follow Illustrations)

Barbara Lewiss

EXCLUSIVE BONUS FOR YOU!

Unlock Your Bonus and Enhance Your Balance Journey!

To further enrich your journey and ensure you're equipped with all the tools needed for success, we're thrilled to offer you an **exclusive bonus.**

Video Demonstrations: Unlock comprehensive video demonstrations of all exercises presented in this book. These guided visuals are meticulously designed to ensure you can accurately and safely follow each movement, significantly enhancing your understanding and execution.

By purchasing this book, you've secured **FREE lifetime access** to these invaluable resources. To claim your bonus, simply turn to the chapter titled **'YOUR BONUS'** and follow the easy instructions laid out for you.

Congratulations once again on embarking on this journey toward better balance and stability. Here's to your continued success!

Warmest regards,
Barbara Lewiss

Table of Contents

Introduction

Understanding Balance: More Than Just Standing Up

Balance is a complex, vital skill that affects every aspect of our daily lives, yet it is often taken for granted until it is compromised. At its core, balance is the ability to maintain the body's center of gravity over its base of support. Whether we're standing still, walking, or performing more dynamic movements, a finely tuned balance system allows us to navigate our environment safely and efficiently.

However, balance is more than just the physical act of standing up. It involves a sophisticated interplay between the visual system (what we see), the vestibular system (the inner ear's role in controlling balance), and proprioception (the sense of our body's position in space). These systems work in harmony, sending constant feedback to the brain to adjust and stabilize our movements.

As we age, changes in these systems can disrupt this harmony, leading to an increased risk of falls and decreased independence. Factors such as muscle weakness, reduced joint flexibility, slower reflexes, and changes in vision or hearing can all contribute to balance decline. Yet, with understanding and practice, much of this decline can be mitigated or even reversed.

This section of the book aims to deepen your understanding of balance — how it works, why it sometimes fails us, and what we can do to strengthen it. By appreciating the complexity of balance, you can better appreciate the exercises and strategies that follow, designed to enhance your stability and confidence in every step you take.

The Importance of Balance as We Age

As we journey through life, our bodies undergo countless changes, many of which can subtly erode our sense of balance. This makes the cultivation and maintenance of good balance an essential aspect of aging gracefully and safely.

Good balance is the cornerstone of active aging, allowing seniors to continue engaging in daily activities, hobbies, and social interactions with confidence and reduced fear of falling.

Falls are a leading cause of injury among older adults, often resulting in a loss of independence, prolonged hospital stays, and in severe cases, life-threatening injuries. However, the repercussions of balance decline extend beyond the physical. The fear of falling can lead to activity avoidance, social isolation, and depression, further diminishing quality of life.

Maintaining or improving balance through targeted exercises not only minimizes the risk of falls but also contributes to overall health and wellbeing. Good balance supports proper posture, which in turn can alleviate or prevent chronic pain conditions. It enhances mobility, making it easier to navigate through different terrains and environments.

Moreover, engaging in balance exercises stimulates cognitive functions, as balance requires continuous, dynamic decision-making processes.

In essence, as we age, balance becomes a critical determinant of our independence and lifestyle quality. Recognizing its importance is the first step toward taking proactive measures to preserve and enhance this vital skill, ensuring that our golden years remain vibrant and fulfilling.

How to Use This Book for Maximum Benefit

This book is designed to be your companion in enhancing balance and ensuring a safer, more active lifestyle as you age. To derive the maximum benefit from it, approach the exercises and advice with a mindset of gradual progress and consistent practice.

Balance, like any skill, improves with time and patience; hence, rushing through the exercises or expecting immediate results may lead to frustration or, worse, injury.

Begin by thoroughly reading the introduction and the first chapter to assess your current balance level. This foundational understanding will guide you in selecting the appropriate starting point within the exercise chapters. Whether you're a beginner, at an intermediate level, or seeking advanced challenges, the book offers tailored plans to suit your needs.

For beginners, it's crucial to start with the exercises listed under "Safe Start: Exercises with Support." These exercises are designed to gently introduce your body to balance training in a secure manner, minimizing the risk of falls. As your confidence and stability improve, progress to the "Building Confidence: Solo Exercises for Stability," which will further challenge and enhance your balance without support.

Intermediates and advanced individuals should still review the beginner exercises to ensure a comprehensive understanding of balance fundamentals. Then, proceed to the exercises and plans designed for your level, always listening to your body and adjusting the intensity as needed.

Incorporate the exercises into your daily routine, aiming for consistency rather than intensity. Consistent, daily practice, even for a few minutes, is more beneficial than sporadic, intense sessions. Utilize the "FAQs on Balance Exercises and Safety" to address common concerns and ensure a safe practice environment.

Finally, engage with the chapters on lifestyle adjustments and from practice to habit to integrate balance-enhancing activities into every aspect of your life.

By following this book's guidance, tracking your progress, and embracing a proactive approach to balance, you'll enjoy the benefits of improved stability, reduced fall risk, and an overall enhanced quality of life as you age.

FAQs on Balance Exercises and Safety

Embarking on a journey to improve balance involves not just dedication and practice, but also awareness and precaution. To ensure that you navigate this path with both confidence and safety, we've compiled a list of frequently asked questions about balance exercises and safety.

This section aims to address your concerns, clarify doubts, and help you make informed decisions about your balance training regimen.

Q: How often should I perform balance exercises?
A: For optimal results, aim to practice balance exercises daily. Consistency is key. Even a short duration of 10 to 15 minutes of focused exercise can lead to significant improvements over time.

Q: Can balance exercises prevent falls?
A: Yes, engaging in regular balance exercises can significantly reduce your risk of falls by improving your stability, strength, and reaction times. These exercises are designed to mimic real-life situations that challenge your balance, preparing your body to better handle them.

Q: Are these exercises safe for everyone?
A: While balance exercises are beneficial for most people, it's important to tailor your exercise routine to your current health status and balance capability. If you have any chronic conditions, mobility issues, or other health concerns, consult with a healthcare professional before starting.

Q: What if I experience discomfort or dizziness while exercising?
A: If you feel dizzy, lightheaded, or experience any discomfort while performing balance exercises, stop immediately. Rest and ensure you're hydrated. If the sensation persists, consult a healthcare provider to rule out any underlying conditions.

Q: What precautions should I take to ensure safety during exercises?
A: Always perform exercises in a safe environment—free of obstacles and with a sturdy support available, such as a chair or a wall. Wear comfortable, non-slip footwear and consider having a partner or caregiver nearby, especially when trying new exercises or if you're prone to dizziness.

Q: Can balance exercises improve my daily activities?

A: Absolutely. Improved balance enhances your overall mobility and confidence in performing daily activities, from walking up stairs to carrying groceries. You'll likely notice a positive impact on your independence and quality of life.

Q: How quickly can I expect to see improvements in my balance?
A: The rate of improvement varies from person to person, depending on factors like initial balance ability, consistency in practice, and overall health. Many individuals begin to notice improvements within a few weeks of regular practice. However, significant and lasting improvements typically require sustained effort over months. It's important to maintain realistic expectations and celebrate small progressions as part of your journey.

Q: Can balance exercises be performed by individuals with a history of joint pain or arthritis?
A: Yes, individuals with joint pain or arthritis can and should engage in balance exercises, but with modifications tailored to their comfort and safety. Low-impact exercises that minimize stress on the joints, such as seated or supported standing exercises, can be particularly beneficial. Consulting with a physiotherapist or healthcare provider can provide personalized advice and adjustments to ensure these exercises support your health without exacerbating pain.

This FAQ section is designed to empower you with the knowledge needed to safely and effectively integrate balance exercises into your life. As you progress through this book, remember that each step you take not only moves you closer to achieving better balance but also contributes to a more active and fulfilling lifestyle.

Chapter 1: Assessing Your Balance

Self-Assessment Tools and Techniques

Understanding your current balance capabilities is essential for tailoring your balance improvement program and tracking progress over time. Here are some straightforward self-assessment tools and techniques you can use at home:

1. **Stance Test**:

   - **How to Perform**: Stand with your feet together and arms crossed over your chest.
   - **Goal**: Maintain this position without swaying or stepping out of place.
   - **Benchmark**: Aim to hold this position for at least 30 seconds. For an additional challenge, try performing the test on a soft surface or with your eyes closed.

2. **Tandem Stand**:

   - **How to Perform**: Place one foot directly in front of the other, heel to toe, and hold the position.
   - **Goal**: Assess and improve balance.
   - **Progression**: Start with eyes open; as confidence increases, perform with eyes closed to enhance difficulty.

3. **Walk and Turn**:

   - **How to Perform**: Mark a straight line on the floor. Walk along it heel-to-toe for 20 steps, turn around, and walk back.
   - **Goal**: Mimic everyday movements to challenge balance and coordination.
   - **Insight**: This dynamic test offers insight into your ability to maintain balance during movement.

4. **One-Leg Stand**:

   - **How to Perform**: Lift one foot a few inches off the ground.
   - **Goal**: Maintain balance on a single leg without support.
   - **Benchmark**: Strive for a 30-second hold on each leg.

By integrating these self-assessment exercises into your routine, not only do you gain a clearer understanding of your balance strengths and weaknesses, but you also actively engage in practices that can enhance your stability.

Repeating these assessments periodically will allow you to measure your improvement concretely and adjust your exercise program to continuously challenge and improve your balance.

Setting Your Balance Baseline

After conducting self-assessment tools and techniques, the next crucial step is to establish your balance baseline. This initial measurement serves as a reference point from which you can monitor your progress and adjust your training accordingly. Here's how to set and understand your balance baseline effectively:

1. **Record Your Results**: After performing the self-assessment exercises, jot down your scores or the duration you were able to maintain each stance. This data forms your personal balance baseline.

2. **Analyze Patterns**: Look for patterns in your assessment results. Are there particular exercises where you struggled more? This can help pinpoint specific areas of weakness that need targeted improvement.

3. **Set Realistic Goals**: Based on your baseline, set achievable goals for improvement. For example, if you held a one-leg stand for 15 seconds, aim to increase this to 25 seconds over the next few weeks.

4. **Consistent Re-evaluation**: Schedule regular reassessments every 2-4 weeks to monitor your progress. Consistent evaluation helps you see improvements, however small, and keeps you motivated.

5. **Adjust Your Plan**: Use the insights gained from your reassessments to refine your balance exercise plan. If you've met or exceeded your goals in certain areas, introduce new exercises to continue challenging yourself.

By establishing a clear balance baseline and regularly revisiting your goals, you create a structured path toward improved stability and reduced fall risk.

Remember, progress in balance training is often gradual and requires patience and persistence. Celebrate every improvement, no matter how small, as a step forward in maintaining independence and enhancing your quality of life.

Understanding and Managing Vertigo During Exercises

Vertigo during exercises can be both a cause and a symptom of balance issues, making it an essential factor to understand and manage for anyone looking to improve their balance.

Vertigo can make balance exercises feel daunting, but with the right knowledge and approach, it can be effectively managed.

1. **Understanding Vertigo**: Vertigo is the sensation of spinning or swaying while you're stationary. It's often caused by issues within the inner ear, which plays a crucial role in maintaining balance. Recognizing the difference between momentary dizziness and vertigo is key to managing it during exercises.

2. **Choose the Right Exercises**: If you experience vertigo, start with low-risk, supported exercises. Activities that involve changing head positions slowly or maintaining a fixed gaze can help in reducing the sensation of spinning. Avoid rapid or extensive head movements initially.

3. **Create a Safe Environment**: Ensure you're exercising in a safe, hazard-free area where you can comfortably sit or lie down if vertigo becomes overwhelming. Having a chair, wall, or another stable object to hold onto can provide additional security.

4. **Focus on Breathing**: Deep, controlled breathing can help mitigate the onset of vertigo by calming the nervous system and reducing stress, which is often a trigger for vertigo episodes. Incorporate mindful breathing into your balance exercises.

5. **Gradual Progression**: As you become more comfortable and experience fewer vertigo symptoms, gradually introduce more challenging exercises. Always listen to your body and progress at a pace that feels safe for you.

6. **Consult a Specialist**: If vertigo is a frequent issue, it's essential to consult with a healthcare professional. They can provide specific exercises to address the underlying causes of your vertigo and recommend a personalized exercise plan.

Understanding and managing vertigo is crucial for safely improving balance through exercises. By starting slow, creating a supportive environment, and knowing when to seek professional advice, you can effectively incorporate balance training into your routine without letting vertigo hold you back.

When to Consult a Professional

While self-assessment tools and techniques are valuable for improving balance, there are instances when consulting a healthcare professional is crucial. Recognizing the signs that indicate the need for professional guidance can ensure that you receive the appropriate care and support to manage balance issues effectively.

Persistent or Worsening Symptoms: If you experience persistent balance problems, dizziness, or vertigo that does not improve with self-managed exercises, it's time to consult a professional. These symptoms can indicate underlying conditions that require medical intervention.

After a Fall: Experiencing a fall can be a sign of significant balance impairment. It's important to seek professional evaluation to understand the causes of the fall and to prevent future incidents. A healthcare provider can assess for injuries and recommend a tailored exercise program.

Increased Frequency of Near Falls: If you find yourself frequently catching yourself to prevent a fall or experiencing more "close calls," it's a sign that your balance may be deteriorating. A professional can help identify specific balance deficits and provide targeted interventions.

Vertigo with Other Symptoms: Vertigo accompanied by symptoms such as hearing loss, tinnitus, or neurological signs like weakness, numbness, or difficulty speaking, should prompt immediate professional consultation. These could be signs of more serious conditions like Meniere's disease or stroke.

Lack of Progress: If you do not see improvement in your balance after consistently following a balance exercise regimen, a healthcare professional can assess your technique, provide feedback, and adjust your exercise plan to better meet your needs.
Choosing the Right Professional: For balance issues, consider consulting a physical therapist specialized in balance and vestibular disorders, an otolaryngologist (ear, nose, and throat doctor), or a neurologist, depending on your symptoms. They can offer diagnostic assessments, personalized exercise plans, and other treatments tailored to your specific condition.

Remember, early intervention by a professional can make a significant difference in managing balance issues, improving your quality of life, and preventing falls. Don't hesitate to reach out for help when needed to ensure you're on the right path to maintaining and improving your balance.

Chapter 2: Beginner Balance Exercises

Safe Start: Exercises with Support

Embarking on a journey to improve your balance begins with a solid foundation. The exercises we present in this section are designed to offer a safe starting point for individuals at the beginning stages of their balance improvement journey.
Recognizing that balance can be a delicate skill to master, especially as we age or recover from health setbacks, these exercises are crafted to provide the support you need while gently challenging your ability to maintain stability.

Using support, such as a chair, wall, or countertop, these exercises aim to reduce the risk of falls and build confidence in your balance capabilities. This approach allows you to focus on the quality of your movements, ensuring proper form and gradual progression in your balance training. By starting with supported exercises, you're not only safeguarding against potential injuries but also laying the groundwork for more advanced balance challenges in the future.

This thoughtful progression is key to developing a sense of security in your balance exercises. It's about acknowledging where you are in your balance journey and taking the necessary steps to move forward safely. As you engage with these exercises, you'll discover the benefits of starting with support, including improved posture, strength, and, most importantly, confidence in your ability to maintain balance in various situations.

Let these exercises be your guide as you begin to explore the realm of balance training. Remember, every step taken with support is a step toward greater independence and stability.

1. Supported Heel Lifts

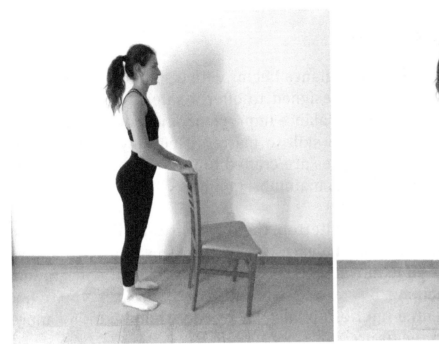 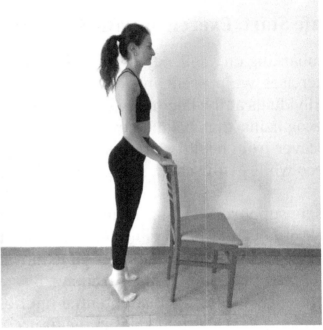

Setup:

1. Stand behind a chair, wall, or countertop for support. Place your feet hip-width apart.
2. Lightly rest your hands on the support structure to ensure stability without leaning your full weight on it.

How To Perform:

1. Slowly lift your heels off the ground, rising onto your toes as high as you can.
2. Hold the position for a count of two.
3. Gently lower your heels back to the floor.

Purpose:
This exercise strengthens the calf muscles, improves ankle stability, and promotes balance by engaging the muscles required for maintaining an upright position.

2. Chair Assisted Side Leg Raise

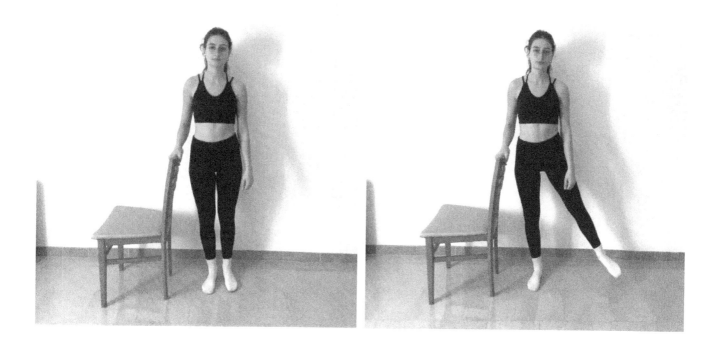

Setup:

1. Stand with a chair on your right side, placing your right hand on the back of the chair for support.
2. Stand straight with your feet placed together, ensuring your body is aligned and upright.

How To Perform:

1. Keeping your left leg straight, slowly lift it to the side as high as comfortably possible without tilting your torso.
2. Pause at the top of the movement for a moment.
3. Slowly lower your leg back to the starting position.

Purpose:
This exercise targets the muscles in the outer thigh and hip, crucial for lateral stability and balance. It also encourages core engagement to maintain an upright posture.

3. Wall Push-Ups

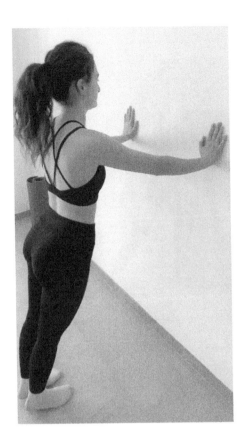 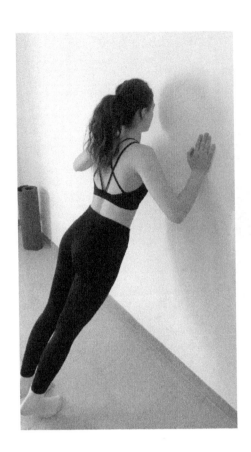

Setup:

1. Face a wall, standing a little further than arm's length away. Feet should be hip-width apart.
2. Place your palms flat against the wall at shoulder height and width.

How To Perform:

1. Bend your elbows to slowly bring your chest toward the wall while keeping your back and legs straight.
2. Push through your hands to extend your arms, returning to the starting position.
3. Ensure the movement is controlled and your core is engaged throughout.

Purpose:
Wall push-ups strengthen the chest, shoulders, and arms, providing upper body strength that supports overall balance and stability. This exercise also engages the core, promoting good posture.

4. Sit to Stand

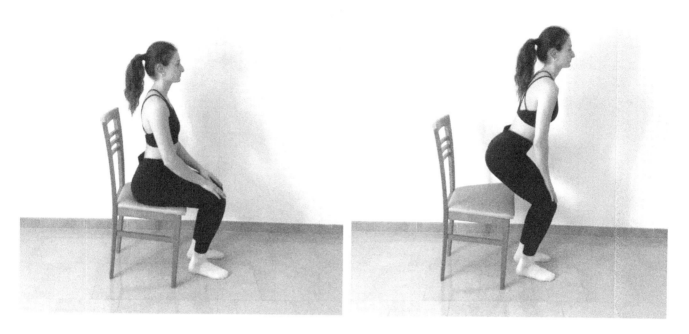

Setup:

1. Begin seated in a sturdy chair without armrests, feet flat on the floor, knees bent at about 90 degrees.
2. Position your feet hip-width apart and slightly back towards the chair.

How To Perform:

1. Lean slightly forward at the hips, keeping your back straight.
2. Press through your heels to stand up, using your leg muscles rather than pushing off with your hands.
3. Once fully standing, pause for a moment to stabilize.
4. Slowly lower yourself back down to the seated position, controlling the movement without collapsing back into the chair.

Purpose:

This exercise strengthens the thighs, buttocks, and core muscles, which are essential for getting up from a seated position, standing, and walking. It also promotes balance and stability through the act of standing up and sitting down.

5. Standing Knee Lifts

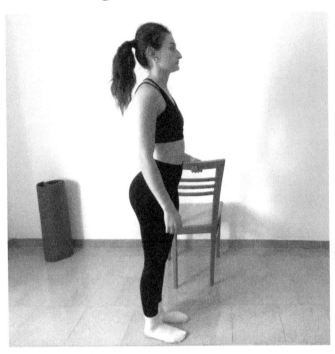 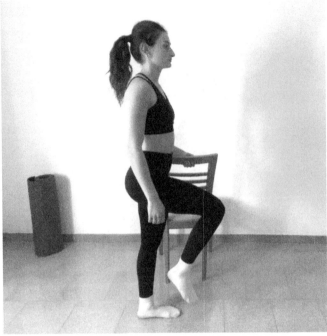

Setup:

1. Stand upright with a chair to your side for balance, if needed.
2. Place your feet hip-width apart, and lightly touch the back of the chair with one hand.

How To Perform:

1. Slowly lift one knee toward your chest, as high as comfortably possible, without leaning backward.
2. Keep the lifted leg in the air for a moment, focusing on balance.
3. Gently lower the foot back to the floor.
4. Alternate legs, performing the lift with the opposite knee.

Purpose:
Standing knee lifts improve balance and stability by strengthening the hip flexors and core muscles. This exercise also encourages coordination and helps maintain the ability to perform daily activities that require lifting the legs, such as climbing stairs.

6. Standing Leg Curls

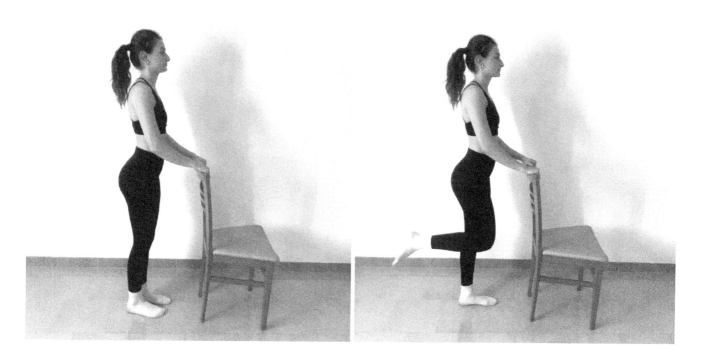

Setup:

1. Stand upright with a chair in front of you, hands lightly resting on the back of the chair for support.
2. Keep your feet hip-width apart and your knees slightly bent.

How To Perform:

1. Curl one leg at the knee, bringing your heel up towards your buttocks as far as possible without moving your thigh.
2. Hold the position briefly at the top of the curl.
3. Slowly lower the foot back to the starting position, keeping the movement controlled.
4. Alternate legs, performing the curl with the opposite leg.

Purpose:

This exercise targets the hamstrings, which are crucial for walking, climbing, and maintaining lower body strength. It helps improve balance by engaging the muscles used in walking and standing activities, promoting overall stability.

7. Standing Hip Extensions

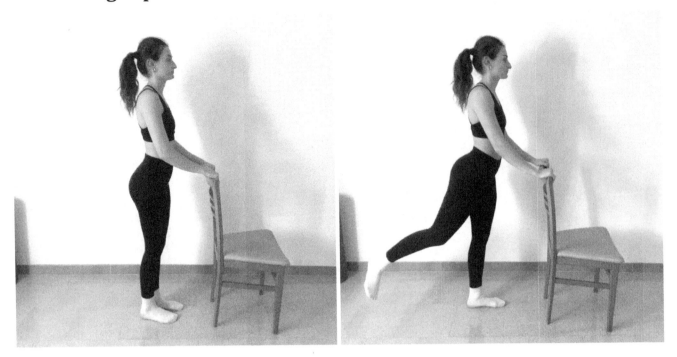

Setup:

1. Stand with your feet hip-width apart, holding onto the back of a chair or a countertop for support.
2. Keep your spine neutral and your core engaged.

How To Perform:

1. Keeping your knee straight, slowly extend one leg back behind you without arching your back.
2. Hold the extension for a few seconds, then gently lower your leg back to the starting position.
3. Alternate legs, performing the exercise with control and without swinging your leg.

Purpose:
Standing hip extensions strengthen the gluteal muscles and the hamstrings, which are crucial for maintaining upright posture, walking, and climbing stairs. This exercise aids in stabilizing the pelvis and improving overall balance during movement.

Elevating Foundations: A Balanced Approach

In this segment, "Elevating Foundations: A Balanced Approach," we transition to a series of exercises that build upon the foundations laid by earlier activities.
These exercises are designed to incrementally increase your balance capabilities, blending both supported and solo exercises to create a comprehensive balance-enhancing routine.

The exercises you'll encounter are crafted to be a step up from the initial supported exercises, offering a balanced mix that challenges your body in new ways. This approach ensures a gradual progression, focusing on developing the core stability, posture, and overall balance necessary for everyday movements and beyond.

Whether you're performing these exercises with or without support, each one aims to strengthen the crucial muscles involved in balance, as well as enhance your mobility and flexibility.
By engaging in these carefully selected exercises, you will further solidify your balance foundation, preparing you for more advanced stability challenges.

8. Seated Toe Taps

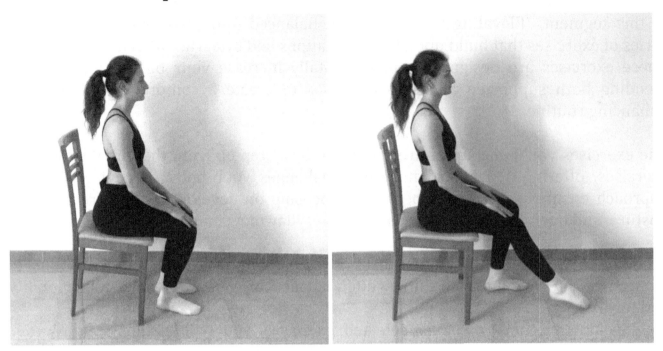

Setup:

1. Sit on a sturdy chair with your back straight and feet flat on the ground.
2. Place your hands on your thighs or the sides of the chair for support.

How To Perform:

1. Lift your right foot off the ground and gently tap the toes on the floor in front of you.
2. Return your right foot to the starting position.
3. Repeat with your left foot, alternating between the right and left for each tap.

Purpose:
This exercise improves lower leg strength and coordination, enhancing your ability to maintain balance while transitioning from sitting to standing positions.

9. Marching in Place

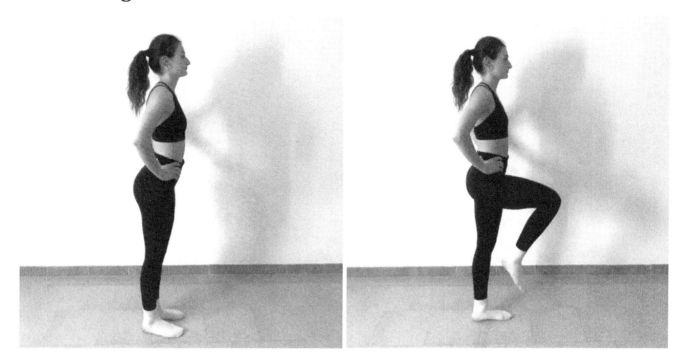

Setup:

1. Stand upright with your feet hip-width apart.
2. Place your hands on your hips or let them hang by your sides for balance.

How To Perform:

1. Lift your right knee towards your chest as high as comfortably possible.
2. Lower your right foot back to the ground.
3. Repeat with your left knee, alternating between the right and left as if marching on the spot.

Purpose:

Marching in place strengthens your hip flexors and core muscles, vital for stabilizing your body during movement and improving overall balance.

10. Hip Circles in Chair

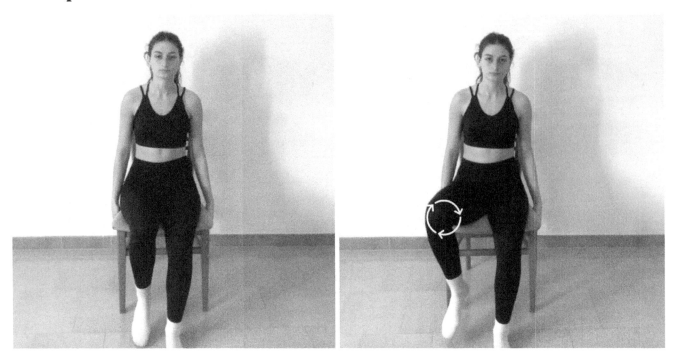

Setup:

1. Sit in a chair with your feet flat on the floor and hands resting on your thighs.
2. Ensure there is enough space around you to move your legs freely.

How To Perform:

1. Lift your right knee slightly and draw a circle in the air with your knee, moving from the hip joint.
2. Complete the circle motion 5 times clockwise and then 5 times counterclockwise.
3. Repeat the same motion with your left knee.

Purpose:
Hip circles enhance hip mobility and flexibility, which are crucial for maintaining balance during various daily activities and preventing falls.

11. Weight Shifts

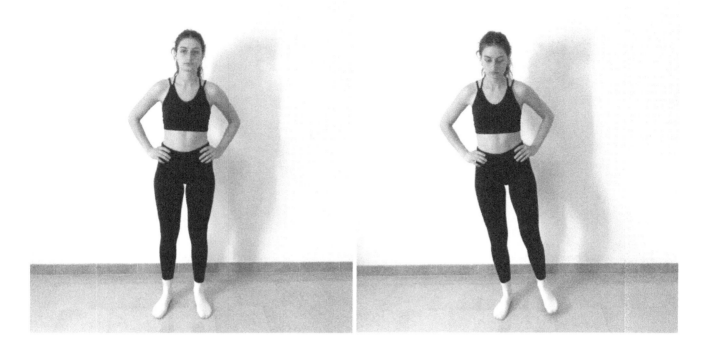

Setup:

1. Stand with your feet hip-width apart, knees slightly bent.
2. Keep your hands on your hips or let them hang by your sides.

How To Perform:

1. Slowly shift your weight onto your right foot, lifting your left foot slightly off the ground.
2. Hold this position for a few seconds, then slowly shift your weight to your left foot, lifting your right foot slightly off the ground.
3. Continue alternating between sides, maintaining control and balance during each shift.

Purpose:
Weight shifts improve your ability to distribute your body weight from one leg to the other, enhancing lateral balance and stability. This exercise is fundamental for walking and standing activities.

12. Toe and Heel Raises

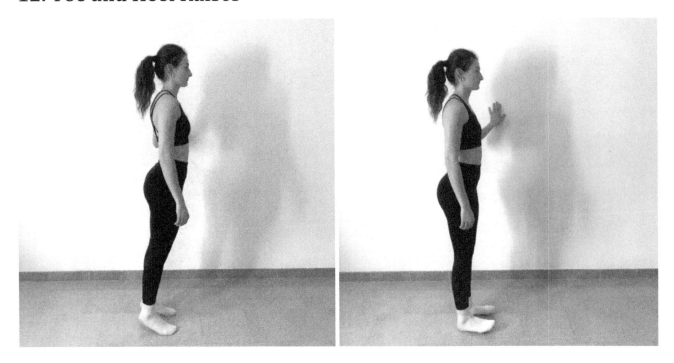

Setup:

1. Stand upright with your feet hip-width apart.
2. Hold onto a chair or wall for support if necessary.

How To Perform:

1. Slowly raise your heels off the ground, coming onto your toes.
2. Hold the position for a few seconds, then slowly lower your heels back to the ground.
3. Next, lift your toes, shifting your weight onto your heels.
4. Hold again for a few seconds before returning to the starting position.

Purpose:

Toe and heel raises strengthen the muscles in your calves and ankles, crucial for walking, climbing stairs, and maintaining an upright posture. This exercise helps prevent falls by improving your forward and backward balance.

13. Shoulder Blade Squeeze

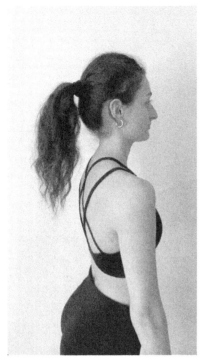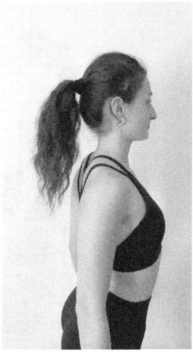

Setup:

1. Stand or sit with your back straight and shoulders relaxed.
2. Place your arms by your sides or on your lap.

How To Perform:

1. Gently pull your shoulder blades towards each other, as if trying to hold a pencil between them.
2. Hold the squeeze for a few seconds, then slowly release and return to the starting position.
3. Repeat the exercise, maintaining a focus on controlled movements and not elevating your shoulders towards your ears.

Purpose:

The shoulder blade squeeze strengthens the muscles around your upper back and shoulders, promoting better posture and upper body stability. A strong upper body supports balance and reduces the risk of upper body strains from falls or sudden movements.

14. Seated Leg Extensions

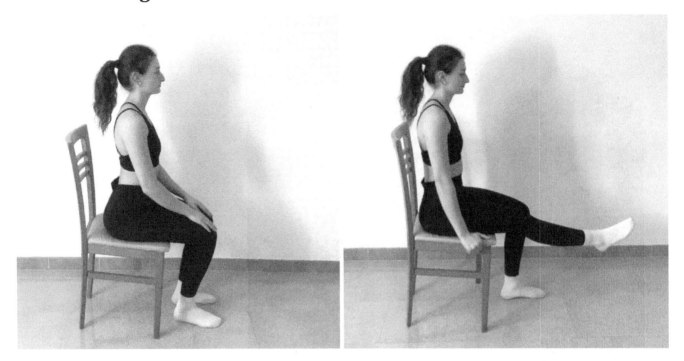

Setup:

1. Sit on a stable chair with your feet flat on the ground and your back straight.
2. Place your hands on the sides of the chair for stability.

How To Perform:

1. Extend one leg at a time, straightening it out in front of you.
2. Hold the extension for a few seconds, then slowly lower your leg back to the starting position.
3. Alternate legs, focusing on a smooth and controlled motion without leaning backward.

Purpose:

Seated leg extensions strengthen the quadriceps, the muscles at the front of your thigh. Strong quadriceps are essential for getting up from a seated position, walking, and climbing stairs. This exercise enhances stability and reduces the risk of knee injuries.

15. Balanced Tandem Stand

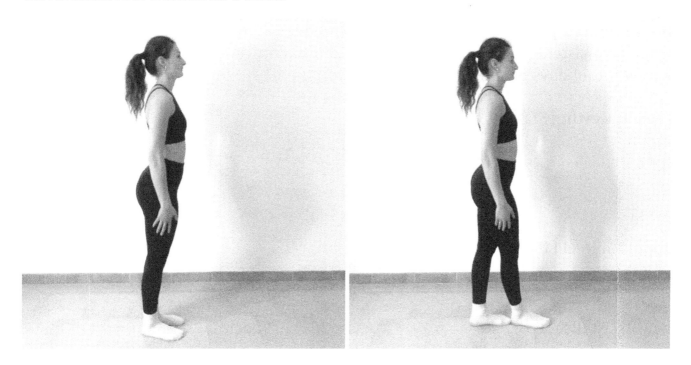

Setup:

1. Stand upright with your feet together and arms at your sides.
2. Choose a focal point ahead to maintain focus and balance.

How To Perform:

1. Place one foot directly in front of the other, heel to toe, as if you are walking on a tightrope.
2. Hold this tandem position for up to 30 seconds, then switch your feet and repeat.
3. Maintain your balance without swaying, using your arms for balance if necessary.

Purpose:
The balanced tandem stand improves your ability to maintain stability on a narrow base of support, mimicking conditions encountered in everyday activities like walking on uneven surfaces. This exercise challenges and improves both static and dynamic balance skills.

4-Week Beginner Balance Improvement Plan

This structured plan is aimed at gradually enhancing your balance and coordination through consistent practice. Here's a detailed breakdown for each week, focusing on three workout days per week.

Week 1: Getting Started

Day 1

Exercise	Page	Sets & Repetitions / Duration
Supported Heel Lifts	p.18	2 sets x 10 reps
Seated Toe Taps	p.26	2 sets x 15 reps
Chair Assisted Side Leg Raise	p.19	2 sets x 10 reps (each side)

Day 2

Exercise	Page	Sets & Repetitions / Duration
Wall Push-Ups	p.20	2 sets x 8 reps
Marching in Place	p.27	2 sets x 20 seconds
Standing Knee Lifts	p.22	2 sets x 10 reps (each side)

Day 3

Exercise	Page	Sets & Repetitions / Duration
Sit to Stand	p.21	2 sets x 8 reps
Hip Circles in Chair	p.28	2 sets x 10 reps (each direction)
Standing Leg Curls	p.23	2 sets x 10 reps (each leg)

Week 2: Building Confidence

Day 1:

Exercise	Page	Sets & Repetitions / Duration
Weight Shifts	p.29	2 sets x 12 reps (each side)
Toe and Heel Raises	p.30	2 sets x 15 reps
Shoulder Blade Squeeze	p.31	2 sets x 12 reps

Day 2:

Exercise	Page	Sets & Repetitions / Duration
Standing Hip Extensions	p.24	2 sets x 10 reps (each leg)
Seated Leg Extensions	p.32	2 sets x 10 reps (each leg)
Balanced Tandem Stand	p.33	2 sets x 20 seconds (each side)

Day 3:

Exercise	Page	Sets & Repetitions / Duration
Seated Leg Extensions	p.32	2 sets x 15 reps (each leg)
Marching in Place	p.27	2 sets x 30 seconds
Shoulder Blade Squeeze	p.31	2 sets x 15 reps

Week 3: Enhancing Stability

Day 1:

Exercise	Page	Sets & Repetitions / Duration
Supported Heel Lifts	p.18	3 sets x 12 reps
Seated Toe Taps	p.26	3 sets x 20 reps
Chair Assisted Side Leg Raise	p.19	3 sets x 12 reps (each side)

Day 2:

Exercise	Page	Sets & Repetitions / Duration
Wall Push-Ups	p.20	3 sets x 10 reps
Marching in Place	p.27	3 sets x 30 seconds
Standing Knee Lifts	p.22	3 sets x 12 reps (each side)

Day 3:

Exercise	Page	Sets & Repetitions / Duration
Sit to Stand	p.21	3 sets x 10 reps
Hip Circles in Chair	p.28	3 sets x 12 reps (each direction)
Standing Leg Curls	p.23	3 sets x 12 reps (each leg)

Week 4: Mastering Balance

Day 1:

Exercise	Page	Sets & Repetitions / Duration
Weight Shifts	p.29	3 sets x 15 reps (each side)
Toe and Heel Raises	p.30	3 sets x 20 reps
Shoulder Blade Squeeze	p.31	3 sets x 15 reps

Day 2:

Exercise	Page	Sets & Repetitions / Duration
Standing Hip Extensions	p.24	3 sets x 12 reps (each leg)
Seated Leg Extensions	p.32	3 sets x 12 reps (each leg)
Balanced Tandem Stand	p.33	3 sets x 30 seconds (each side)

Day 3:

Exercise	Page	Sets & Repetitions / Duration
Hip Circles in Chair	p.28	3 sets x 15 reps (each direction)
Standing Hip Extensions	p.24	3 sets x 15 reps (each leg)
Balanced Tandem Stand	p.33	3 sets x 40 seconds (each side)

Ensure to rest adequately between sets and listen to your body, adjusting the intensity as needed.
Consistency and gradual progression are key to improving balance and stability through these exercises.

Chapter 3: Intermediate Balance Challenges

Elevating Your Balance: Intermediate Exercises

The "Intermediate Balance Challenges" are designed to elevate your balance to new heights, pushing the boundaries of what you've achieved so far.
Here, we focus on refining your skills, enhancing your stability, and building the confidence needed to tackle everyday activities with greater ease and safety.

This section of the book introduces a series of intermediate exercises that are carefully curated to challenge your balance system further. While the beginner exercises laid the foundation, these intermediate activities will test your balance under slightly more demanding conditions, encouraging your body and mind to adapt and grow stronger together.

Whether it's performing side leg lifts with your eyes closed, mastering the art of walking on a soft cushion, or executing precise movements along a line, each exercise is a step towards achieving a more stable and confident you.

As you progress through these exercises, remember that balance is not just about physical strength; it's about coordination, focus, and the ability to control your body in various situations. The dynamic movements included in this chapter, such as grapevine walking and rotational reaches, are designed to mimic everyday scenarios, helping you build the kind of balance that not only prevents falls but also enriches your daily life with fluid, effortless motion.

Approach these intermediate challenges with an open mind and a willingness to push yourself, but always within the limits of safety and comfort. Remember, improvement comes with practice and patience. Let's elevate your balance, step by step, towards greater stability and confidence.

1. Side Leg Lifts with Eyes Closed

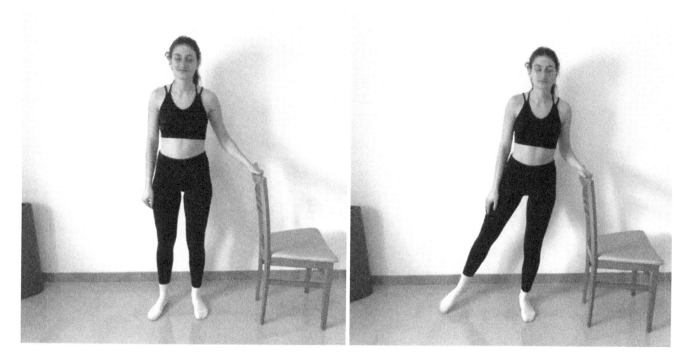

Setup:

1. Stand upright next to a chair or a wall for support.
2. Position your feet hip-width apart.
3. Lightly touch the chair or wall with one hand for stability.

How To Perform:

1. Transfer your weight to one leg, keeping a slight bend in the supporting knee.
2. Slowly lift the opposite leg to the side, keeping your foot flexed and your body straight.
3. Close your eyes and hold the position for a few seconds.
4. Lower your leg back to the starting position.
5. Repeat the exercise on the other side.

Purpose:
This exercise enhances your balance by removing visual cues, forcing your body to rely more on the vestibular and proprioceptive systems for stability. It strengthens the hip abductors and improves your ability to maintain balance in situations where visibility is compromised.

2. Single Leg Stance with Soft Cushion

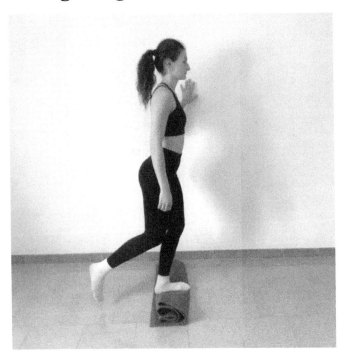

Setup:

1. Place a soft cushion or a folded towel on the floor.
2. Stand next to a chair or a wall for support if needed.

How To Perform:

1. Step onto the cushion with one foot, finding your balance.
2. Lift your opposite foot off the ground, maintaining a slight bend in your standing leg.
3. Hold the position, focusing on stabilizing your body.
4. Switch legs and repeat the exercise.

Purpose:
Standing on a soft surface challenges your balance by creating instability. This exercise strengthens the muscles and joints in your lower body and trains your proprioceptive system, enhancing your ability to balance on uneven surfaces.

3. Tandem Walk Along a Line

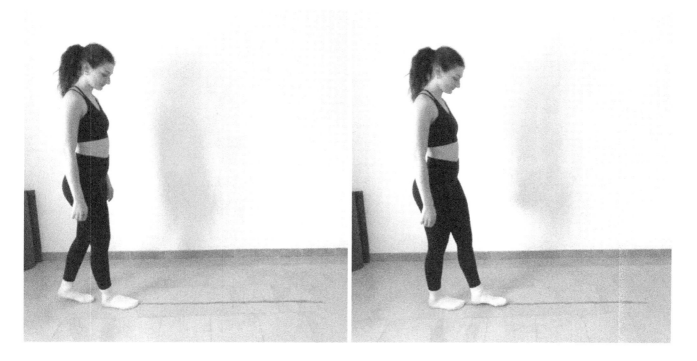

Setup:

1. Find a straight line on the floor or create one with tape.
2. Stand at one end of the line with your feet together.

How To Perform:

1. Place the heel of one foot directly in front of the toes of your other foot as if walking on a tightrope.
2. Walk forward along the line, placing one foot directly in front of the other.
3. Keep your arms out to the sides for balance.
4. Focus on a fixed point ahead to help maintain balance.
5. Walk the length of the line, then turn around and walk back.

Purpose:

This exercise mimics situations where precise foot placement is required, improving your dynamic balance and coordination. It strengthens the muscles used for walking and promotes the integration of visual, vestibular, and proprioceptive inputs for better balance control.

4. Standing on One Leg

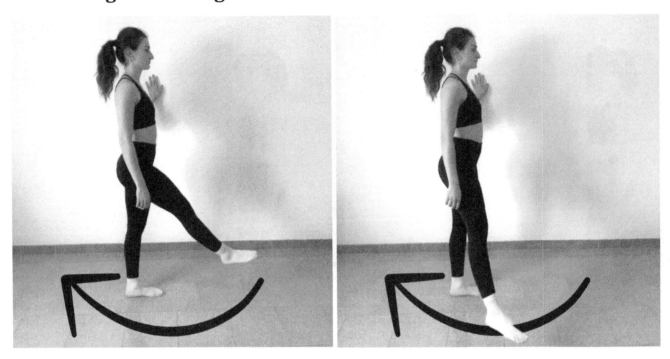

Setup:

1. Stand upright with your feet hip-width apart next to a stable surface if support is needed.
2. Shift your weight to one leg, preparing to lift the other.

How To Perform:

1. Lift the non-supporting leg slightly off the ground, finding your balance.
2. Extend the lifted leg forward (12 o'clock), then to the side (3 o'clock for the right leg, 9 o'clock for the left), and finally slightly behind you (6 o'clock), mimicking the hands of a clock.
3. Keep your supporting leg slightly bent at the knee during the movements.

Purpose: This exercise improves balance and stability by strengthening the lower body muscles and increasing ankle stability. It also enhances coordination and spatial awareness by requiring controlled movements in multiple directions.

5. Sit-to-Stand without Hands

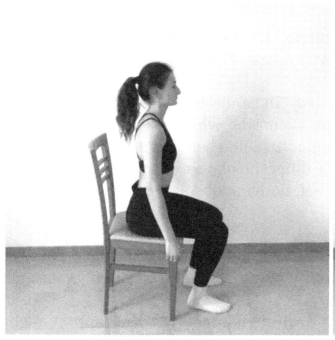 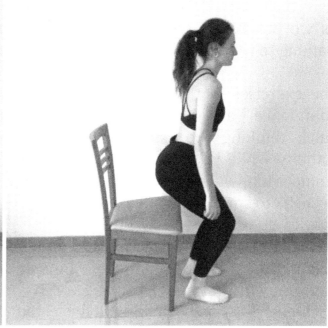

Setup:

1. Begin seated in a sturdy chair without armrests, feet flat on the floor, and knees bent at a 90-degree angle.
2. Position your feet hip-width apart.

How To Perform:

1. Lean slightly forward and push through your heels to stand up, using your leg strength rather than your hands. Close your eyes to make the exercise more effective.
2. Slowly lower yourself back into the chair, controlling the movement and without using your hands for assistance.
3. Repeat the movement, focusing on smooth transitions between sitting and standing.

Purpose: This exercise strengthens the quadriceps, hamstrings, and gluteal muscles, crucial for everyday movements like standing up from a chair or toilet. It promotes lower body strength and endurance, improving balance and reducing the risk of falls.

Dynamic Movements for Everyday Confidence

As we progress into more dynamic movements, it's time to elevate your balance training to reflect the unpredictability of everyday activities.

The exercises in the upcoming sections, titled "Dynamic Movements for Everyday Confidence," are designed to mimic real-life scenarios where balance, agility, and quick thinking are essential. These movements will challenge you to maintain stability while your body navigates through different planes of motion, just as you would when walking through a crowded street, dodging obstacles, or simply turning to speak to someone while standing.

Incorporating these exercises into your routine will not only enhance your physical balance but also build confidence in your ability to move freely and safely in various environments.
Each exercise has been carefully selected to push the boundaries of what you might consider achievable, encouraging your body to adapt and strengthen in new ways.

By practicing these dynamic movements, you'll be better equipped to handle the complexities of everyday life, reducing the risk of falls and increasing your overall mobility and independence.

Remember, the goal here is not perfection but progress. As you embrace these challenges, you'll discover newfound strength and stability that will serve you well beyond your workout sessions. Let's move with purpose, embrace the unexpected, and build a foundation of confidence that will carry you through each day with ease.

6. Grapevine Walking

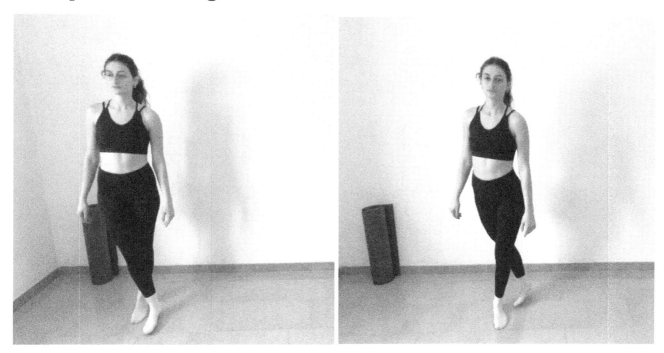

Setup:

1. Stand with your feet hip-width apart in an open space where you can take at least 8-10 steps to your side.
2. Ensure there's nothing in your path that you could trip over.

How To Perform:

1. Start by crossing your right foot over your left.
2. Step out to the left with your left foot.
3. Cross your right foot behind your left.
4. Continue this pattern for 8-10 steps, then switch directions and repeat the sequence with your left foot crossing over and behind the right.
5. Keep your arms out to the sides or on your hips for balance.

Purpose:
This exercise improves lateral movement coordination, agility, and balance. It helps simulate real-life movements, such as navigating through crowded spaces, enhancing your ability to maintain balance while changing directions.

7. Backward Walking

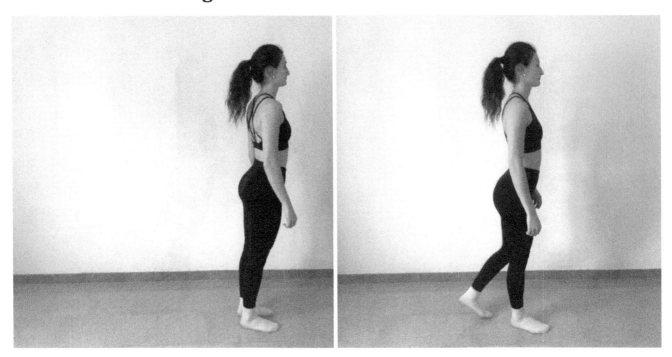

Setup:

1. Find a clear, straight path where you can safely walk backward for at least 10-15 steps.
2. Remove any potential tripping hazards from your path.

How To Perform:

1. Stand with your feet hip-width apart, shoulders relaxed, and looking straight ahead.
2. Take a small step backward with your right foot.
3. Follow with your left foot, continuing to step backward in a controlled manner.
4. Keep your posture upright, and use your arms for balance as needed.
5. After 10-15 steps, stop, turn around, and repeat if space allows.

Purpose:
Backward walking strengthens the leg muscles differently than forward walking or running. It challenges your balance and coordination by changing your usual movement pattern, improving proprioception and reducing the risk of falls by enhancing your ability to react to unexpected changes in terrain or direction.

8. Toe-to-Heel Walks

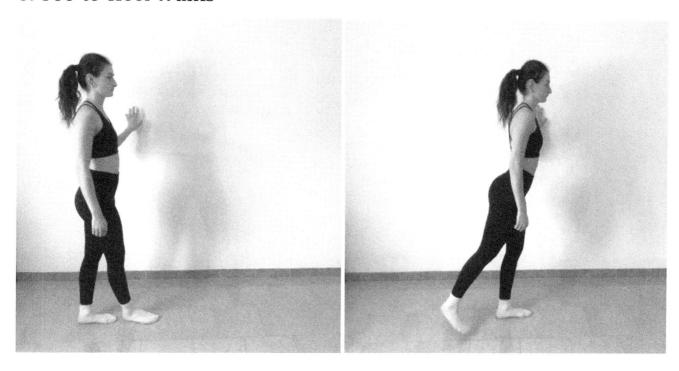

Setup:

1. Clear a straight path where you can safely walk in a straight line for 10-15 steps.
2. If needed, have a wall or sturdy furniture nearby for light support.

How To Perform:

1. Stand with your feet together, looking straight ahead.
2. Place the heel of your right foot directly in front of the toes of your left foot, touching or almost touching.
3. Shift your weight forward onto your right foot.
4. Now place the heel of your left foot directly in front of the toes of your right foot.
5. Continue this heel-to-toe pattern, walking in a straight line for 10-15 steps.
6. Focus on maintaining a straight line and keeping your balance with each step.

Purpose:
This exercise enhances your ability to maintain balance while moving in a controlled, linear fashion. It mimics situations where you need precise foot placement, such as walking along narrow paths or in crowded areas. It improves coordination between your lower body muscles and your visual system, crucial for preventing falls.

9. Side-Stepping with Arm Swings

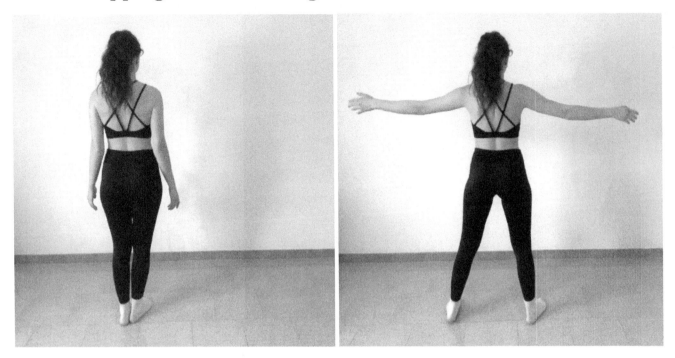

Setup:

1. Stand with your feet hip-width apart in a clear space where you can move side to side.
2. Ensure there's enough room to take 8-10 side steps in either direction.

How To Perform:

1. Begin by stepping to the right with your right foot.
2. Follow with your left foot, bringing it to meet your right.
3. As you step, swing your arms naturally at your sides.
4. Continue for 8-10 steps to the right, then switch directions and repeat to the left.
5. Keep your movements controlled and your posture upright.

Purpose:
This exercise promotes lateral balance and coordination, vital for navigating everyday environments and avoiding falls. The arm swings add an element of upper body coordination, simulating natural walking movements and enhancing overall stability.

10. Standing Marches with High Knees

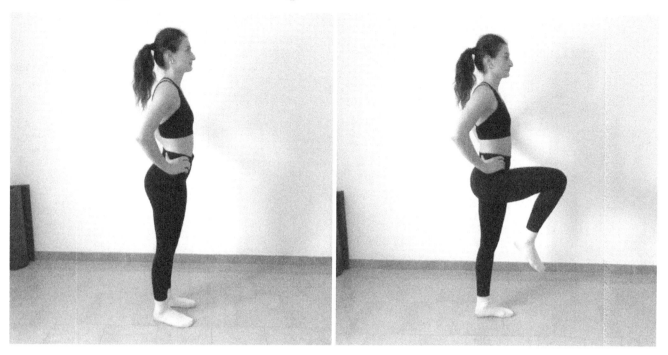

Setup:

1. Stand straight with your feet hip-width apart.
2. Place your hands on your hips or let them hang by your sides.

How To Perform:

1. Lift your right knee as high as you comfortably can, aiming for hip level.
2. Lower your right foot back to the ground and repeat with your left knee.
3. Continue alternating legs, mimicking a marching motion.
4. If you need more balance, raise your arms out to the sides.
5. Perform this marching action for 30 seconds to 1 minute.

Purpose:
This exercise strengthens your hip flexors and thighs, improving your ability to lift your legs and maintain balance when walking or climbing stairs. High knees also engage your core, enhancing stability and posture during dynamic movements.

11. Rotational Reaches

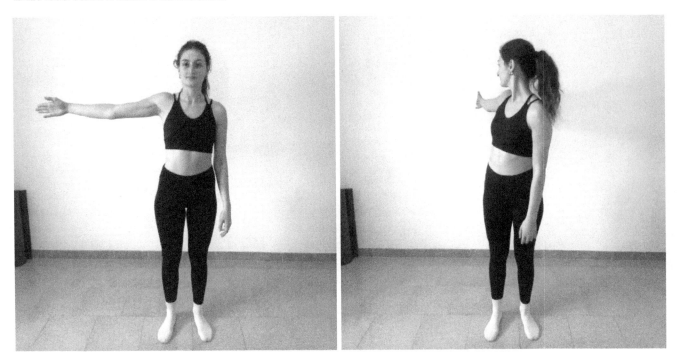

Setup:

1. Stand with feet shoulder-width apart, knees slightly bent.
2. Start with your arms at your sides or on your hips.

How To Perform:

1. Extend your right arm and rotate your torso to the right, reaching as far as comfortable either to the side or up at an angle.
2. Return to the starting position and repeat with your left arm, rotating to the left.
3. Keep your movements fluid and controlled, focusing on the rotation of your waist.
4. Alternate sides for 10-12 repetitions on each side.
5. Ensure your feet remain planted and adjust your stance for balance as you rotate.

Purpose:

This exercise enhances core strength and flexibility, crucial for maintaining balance during rotational movements encountered in daily activities. It trains your body to coordinate movements between the upper and lower halves, improving overall stability and reducing the risk of falls when reaching or turning.

4-Week Intermediate Balance Improvement Plan

This intermediate plan is designed to elevate your balance through targeted exercises over four weeks. Each week, you'll engage in four days of training, incorporating exercises from both the "Elevating Your Balance: Intermediate Exercises" and "Dynamic Movements for Everyday Confidence" sections. Remember, quality over quantity; focus on form and control.

Week 1: Building the Basics

Day 1:

Exercise	Page	Sets & Repetitions / Duration
Side Leg Lifts with Eyes Closed	p.39	2 sets x 10 reps per side
Single Leg Stance with Soft Cushion	p.40	2 sets x 30 seconds per leg
Grapevine Walking	p.45	3 sets x 10 steps each direction

Day 2:

Exercise	Page	Sets & Repetitions / Duration
Tandem Walk Along a Line	p.41	3 sets x 1 minute
Standing on One Leg	p.42	2 sets x 5 reaches per leg
Backward Walking	p.46	3 sets x 1 minute

Day 3:

Exercise	Page	Sets & Repetitions / Duration
Sit-to-Stand without Hands	p.43	2 sets x 10 reps
Toe-to-Heel Walks	p.47	3 sets x 1 minute
Standing Marches with High Knees	p.49	2 sets x 30 seconds

Day 4:

Exercise	Page	Sets & Repetitions / Duration
Side Leg Lifts with Eyes Closed	p.39	3 sets x 10 reps per side
Rotational Reaches	p.50	2 sets x 10 reps each direction
Side-Stepping with Arm Swings	p.48	2 sets x 10 steps each direction

Week 2: Enhancing Stability

Day 1:

Exercise	Page	Sets & Repetitions / Duration
Side Leg Lifts with Eyes Closed	p.39	3 sets x 12 reps per side
Grapevine Walking	p.45	3 sets x 12 steps each direction
Standing Marches with High Knees	p.49	2 sets x 40 seconds

Day 2:

Exercise	Page	Sets & Repetitions / Duration
Single Leg Stance with Soft Cushion	p.40	3 sets x 40 seconds per leg
Tandem Walk Along a Line	p.41	4 sets x 1 minute
Rotational Reaches	p.50	3 sets x 12 reps each direction

Day 3:

Exercise	Page	Sets & Repetitions / Duration
Standing on One Leg	p.42	3 sets x 6 reaches per leg
Toe-to-Heel Walks	p.47	4 sets x 1 minute
Sit-to-Stand without Hands	p.43	3 sets x 12 reps

Day 4:

Exercise	Page	Sets & Repetitions / Duration
Grapevine Walking	p.45	4 sets x 12 steps each direction
Backward Walking	p.46	4 sets x 1 minute
Side-Stepping with Arm Swings	p.48	3 sets x 12 steps each direction

Week 3: Advanced Coordination

Day 1:

Exercise	Page	Sets & Repetitions / Duration
Grapevine Walking	p.45	3 sets x 15 steps each direction
Toe-to-Heel Walks	p.47	4 sets x 1.5 minutes
Sit-to-Stand without Hands	p.43	4 sets x 12 reps

Day 2:

Exercise	Page	Sets & Repetitions / Duration
Side Leg Lifts with Eyes Closed	p.39	3 sets x 15 reps per side
Rotational Reaches	p.50	3 sets x 15 reps each direction
Standing Marches with High Knees	p.49	3 sets x 50 seconds

Day 3:

Exercise	Page	Sets & Repetitions / Duration
Single Leg Stance with Soft Cushion	p.40	3 sets x 50 seconds per leg
Tandem Walk Along a Line	p.41	4 sets x 1.5 minutes
Standing on One Leg	p.42	3 sets x 7 reaches per leg

Day 4:

Exercise	Page	Sets & Repetitions / Duration
Sit-to-Stand without Hands	p.43	3 sets x 15 reps
Backward Walking	p.46	4 sets x 1.5 minutes
Side-Stepping with Arm Swings	p.48	3 sets x 15 steps each direction

Week 4: Mastery and Integration

Day 1:

Exercise	Page	Sets & Repetitions / Duration
Side Leg Lifts with Eyes Closed	p.39	4 sets x 15 reps per side
Grapevine Walking	p.45	4 sets x 15 steps each direction
Rotational Reaches	p.50	4 sets x 15 reps each direction

Day 2:

Exercise	Page	Sets & Repetitions / Duration
Standing on One Leg	p.42	4 sets x 8 reaches per leg
Single Leg Stance with Soft Cushion	p.40	4 sets x 60 seconds per leg
Toe-to-Heel Walks	p.47	5 sets x 1.5 minutes

Day 3:

Exercise	Page	Sets & Repetitions / Duration
Tandem Walk Along a Line	p.41	5 sets x 2 minutes
Sit-to-Stand without Hands	p.43	4 sets x 15 reps
Backward Walking	p.46	5 sets x 1.5 minutes

Day 4:

Exercise	Page	Sets & Repetitions / Duration
Side-Stepping with Arm Swings	p.48	4 sets x 15 steps each direction
Standing Marches with High Knees	p.49	4 sets x 60 seconds
Side Leg Lifts with Eyes Closed	p.39	4 sets x 15 reps per side

This plan is designed to progressively challenge and improve your balance over 4 weeks. Always ensure to perform these exercises in a safe environment and listen to your body, adjusting the intensity as needed.

This plan is designed to progressively challenge and improve your balance over 4 weeks. Always ensure to perform these exercises in a safe environment and listen to your body, adjusting the intensity as needed.

Chapter 4: Advanced Balance Mastery

Achieving Balance Mastery: Advanced Techniques

As you embark on the journey of achieving balance mastery, this section of our book is designed to elevate your skills to an advanced level. "Achieving Balance Mastery: Advanced Techniques" introduces you to a collection of exercises that challenge your balance, coordination, and overall body strength in more complex and demanding ways than ever before.

These exercises are not just about standing on one leg or walking in a straight line; they incorporate elements of strength training, flexibility, and mindful movement to truly test and enhance your equilibrium.

As we delve into advanced balance training, we encourage you to approach these exercises with patience and persistence. The techniques outlined here are meant to push your limits, improve your proprioception, and refine your ability to maintain stability in dynamic and challenging scenarios. Whether it's mastering the Single-Leg Squat, finding your center in the Yoga Tree Pose without support, or engaging in the controlled movement of the Pilates Teaser, each exercise has been carefully selected to contribute to your balance mastery.

Remember, safety should always be your top priority. Ensure that you have a clear space to practice, and consider having a spotter or support nearby, especially when trying these exercises for the first time.
With dedication and practice, you'll not only enhance your balance but also gain a deeper connection between your mind and body, allowing for graceful, confident, and secure movement through all walks of life.

Let's embark on this advanced journey together, pushing boundaries and reaching new heights in balance mastery.

1. Lunges with Arm Lifts

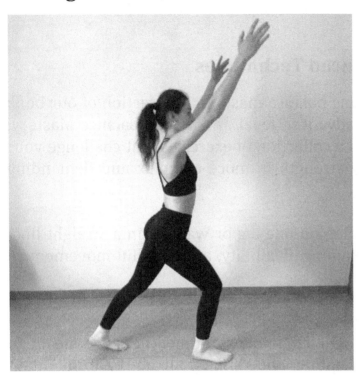

Setup:

1. Stand with your feet together, arms at your sides.
2. Choose a point in front of you to focus on maintaining balance.

How To Perform:

1. Take a step forward with one leg, lowering your hips.
2. As you lunge, lift your arms straight up above your head.
3. Push back up to the starting position, lowering your arms back to your sides.
4. Alternate legs and repeat the exercise.

Purpose:

This exercise integrates upper and lower body movements to enhance overall balance and stability. Lunges strengthen the legs and improve flexibility in the hips, while arm lifts increase shoulder stability and engage the core, promoting a more balanced posture and movement.

2. Yoga Tree Pose without Support

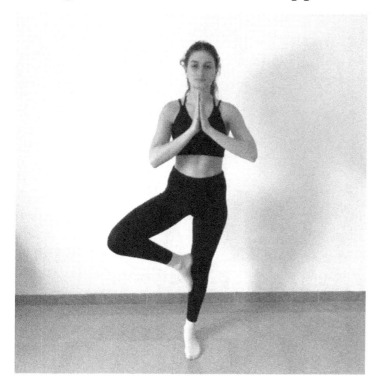

Setup:

1. Stand straight with your arms at your sides and feet together.
2. Shift your weight slightly onto your left foot.

How To Perform:

1. Bend your right knee and place the sole of your right foot on the inner thigh of your left leg, above the knee.
2. Ensure your pelvis is in a neutral position, and your standing leg is straight.
3. Bring your hands together in a prayer position at your chest or raise them above your head.
4. Hold the pose while focusing on a fixed point in front of you to maintain balance.
5. Release gently and switch to the other leg.

Purpose:
This pose improves balance and stability, strengthens the thighs, calves, ankles, and spine, and promotes mental and physical equilibrium.

3. Pilates Teaser

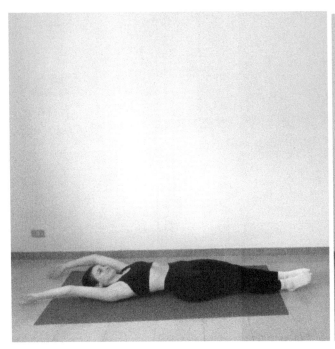 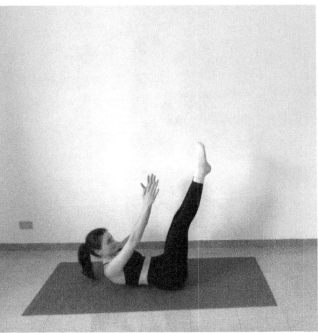

Setup:

1. Lie flat on your back on a mat, legs extended, and arms overhead.
2. Engage your core by pulling your navel towards your spine.

How To Perform:

1. Inhale, and as you exhale, simultaneously lift your legs and upper body off the mat, reaching your hands towards your toes.
2. Your body should form a V shape at the top of the movement.
3. Hold this position briefly, keeping your core engaged and your spine straight.
4. Slowly lower yourself back to the starting position.
5. Repeat the movement while maintaining fluid and controlled motions.

Purpose:
The Pilates Teaser is a comprehensive exercise that strengthens the core, improves balance and posture, and enhances coordination and flexibility.

4. Advanced Tandem Walk with Obstacles

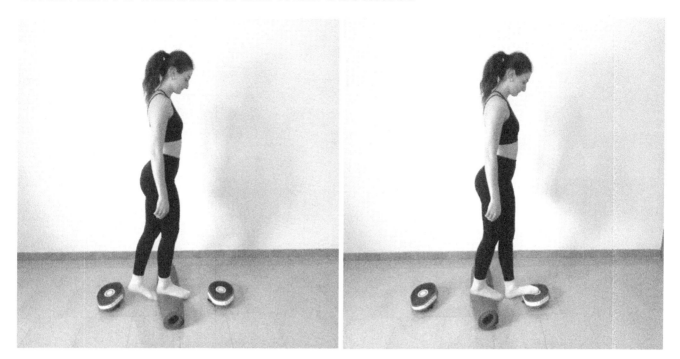

Setup:

1. Place several soft obstacles on the ground in a straight line, such as cushions or foam blocks.
2. Stand at one end of the obstacle line, preparing to walk forward.

How To Perform:

1. Begin by placing one foot directly in front of the other, heel to toe, as if walking on a tightrope.
2. Carefully step over each obstacle, maintaining the heel-to-toe tandem position throughout the walk.
3. Focus on keeping your balance as you navigate the obstacles, using your arms for added stability.
4. Once you reach the end, turn around and repeat the walk back to the starting position.

Purpose:

This exercise challenges your dynamic balance and coordination by adding complexity to the traditional tandem walk. It simulates real-life scenarios where you must navigate uneven terrain or obstacles, enhancing your ability to prevent falls.

5. Single Leg Juggling

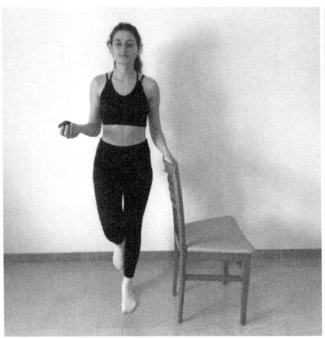 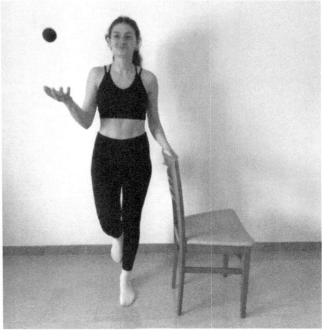

Setup:

1. Begin by standing near a chair or wall for support, if necessary. Ensure you have enough space around you to move freely without knocking into objects.
2. Lift your right foot and place it against your left calf, ensuring your weight is firmly on your left leg.
3. In your left hand, hold a small, lightweight ball that is easy to catch and throw.

How To Perform:

1. Find your balance on your left leg. Once stabilized, start tossing the ball gently into the air with your left hand, aiming for a height that is comfortable for you to catch.
2. Continue juggling the ball for a series of tosses, then switch to balancing on your right leg and juggling with your right hand.

Purpose:
The Single Leg Juggling exercise is designed to significantly improve your body's coordination, balance, and focus. By engaging in this activity, you're not only challenging your physical balance by standing on one leg, but you're also enhancing your hand-eye coordination through the act of juggling.

6. Single-Leg Deadlift

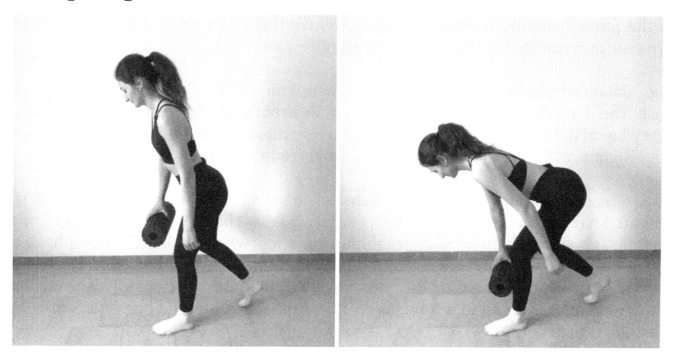

Setup:

1. Stand upright with your feet hip-width apart, holding a lightweight dumbbell in your right hand.
2. Shift your weight onto your left leg.

How To Perform:

1. Keeping a slight bend in your left knee, hinge forward at the hips, extending your right leg straight behind you for balance.
2. Lower the dumbbell towards the ground, keeping it close to your leg, as your torso comes parallel to the floor.
3. Use your left hamstring and glute to pull yourself back to the starting position, keeping your back straight throughout the movement.
4. Repeat the movement, then switch sides.

Purpose:
The Single-Leg Deadlift is a powerful exercise for improving balance, coordination, and strength in the lower back, glutes, and hamstrings. It also enhances stability in the standing leg, contributing to better balance in everyday movements.

Balance in Motion: Integrating Movement with Stability

In the pursuit of advanced balance mastery, we transition from static exercises to dynamic movements that challenge your stability in motion.

The "Balance in Motion: Integrating Movement with Stability" section is designed to push the boundaries of your balance by incorporating movements that mimic everyday activities and sports. These exercises will not only enhance your stability but also improve your agility, coordination, and reaction times.

As we age, our ability to quickly adapt to changing environments and react to potential hazards becomes crucial for preventing falls. The exercises included in this section are selected to simulate real-life scenarios where balance, strength, and cognitive awareness converge. From the fluid movements of Tai Chi, which focus on gentle, controlled motions, to the more lively and rhythmic steps of dance, each activity is tailored to build a foundation that supports a more active and confident lifestyle.

Whether you're navigating uneven terrain, quickly changing direction, or maintaining your center of gravity during complex movements, the skills developed here will serve you in countless situations. By integrating movement with stability, you'll not only safeguard against falls but also move with greater ease and confidence in your daily life.

Prepare to engage your entire body and mind as we embark on this journey of balance in motion.
Let's embrace the challenge, enjoy the process, and celebrate the progress as we work towards achieving balance mastery together.

7. Tai Chi Movements

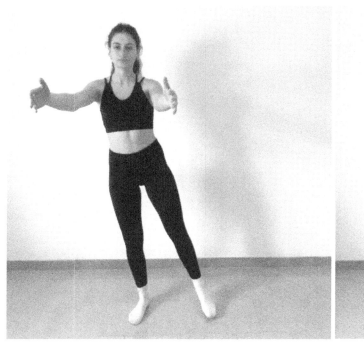 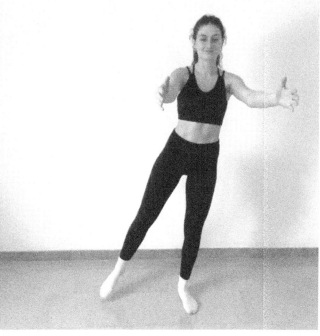

Setup:

1. Find a quiet, open space with enough room to move freely.
2. Stand with your feet shoulder-width apart, knees slightly bent.
3. Relax your shoulders and let your arms hang loosely by your sides.

How To Perform:

1. Begin with the basic Tai Chi posture: Shift your weight to your right leg, step out with your left leg, and gently lift your arms in front of you as if holding a ball.
2. Slowly transfer your weight from one leg to the other, moving your arms in a flowing motion, mirroring the movement of your legs.
3. Focus on maintaining a slow, continuous movement, coordinating your breath with each movement.

Purpose:

Tai Chi movements are designed to improve balance and stability by enhancing proprioception and coordination. The gentle, flowing movements increase flexibility and strength, particularly in the lower body, essential for maintaining balance.

Practicing Tai Chi can also reduce stress and improve mental focus, contributing to better balance awareness and control.

8. Cross-body Toe Touch

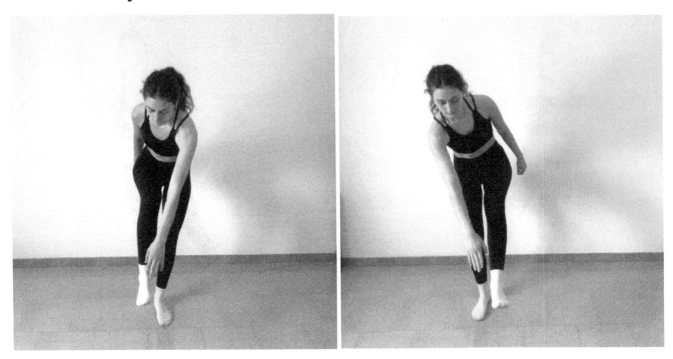

Setup:

1. Begin by standing in an upright position with your feet hip-width apart. Ensure your shoulders are relaxed and down, away from your ears.
2. Engage your core muscles lightly to maintain a strong, stable posture throughout the exercise.

How To Perform:

1. Start by slightly lifting your left foot off the ground to find your balance.
2. Lean forward at your hips, bending slightly at the knees if needed, and reach down across your body with your right hand to touch the toes of your left foot.
3. Slowly return to the starting upright position, maintaining control and balance throughout the movement. Repeat the movement, this time slightly lifting your right foot and reaching down with your left hand to touch the toes of your right foot.

Purpose:
The Cross-body Toe Touch exercise is a dynamic movement designed to enhance balance, flexibility, and coordination. By reaching across the body to touch the opposite foot, you engage multiple muscle groups, including those in the core, lower back, and legs, which are crucial for maintaining balance and stability.

9. Skater Hops

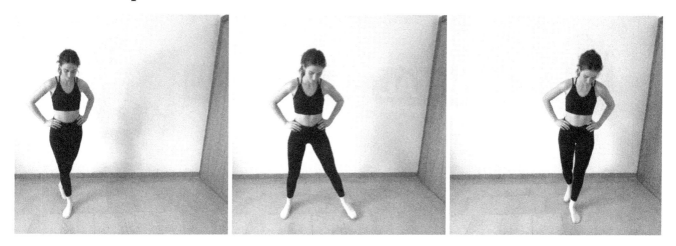

Setup:

1. Clear a space that allows for lateral movement.
2. Stand with your feet hip-width apart, knees slightly bent, ready to move side-to-side.

How To Perform:

1. Push off with your right foot, hopping to your left. Land on your left foot with your right leg behind your left ankle, mimicking a skating movement.
2. Push off with your left foot, hopping to your right, landing on your right foot with your left leg behind your right ankle.
3. Continue these side-to-side hops, maintaining a fluid and controlled motion.

Purpose:

Skater hops improve dynamic balance and lateral stability, crucial for navigating uneven surfaces and making quick turns.

This exercise strengthens the leg muscles, particularly the glutes and quads, which play a significant role in balance.

The coordination required for skater hops enhances neuromuscular control, making it easier to recover balance when destabilized.

10. Cone Taps

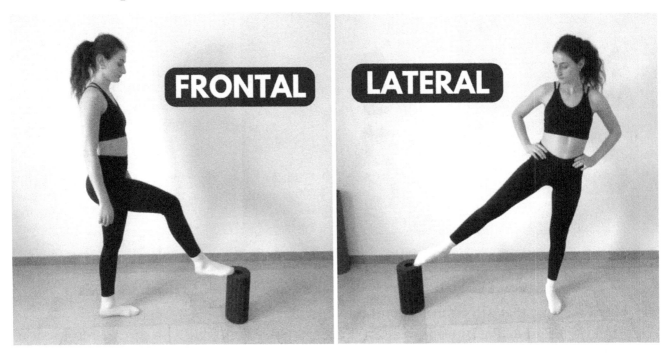

FRONTAL   LATERAL

Setup:

1. Place a cone or a similar object on the ground in front of you and to the side, within easy reach.
2. Stand with your feet hip-width apart, directly in front of the cone.

How To Perform:

1. Shift your weight to your left leg, and with your right foot, gently tap the top of the cone in front of you, then return to the starting position.
2. Next, tap the cone to your right side with the same foot, returning to the starting position after each tap.
3. Alternate between forward and lateral taps, maintaining a steady rhythm and balance on your standing leg.

Purpose:
Cone taps enhance coordination and agility, requiring precise movements while maintaining balance on one leg.This exercise strengthens the stabilizing muscles in the ankles, knees, and hips, which are vital for balance and preventing falls.
Improving lateral movement is essential for navigating everyday environments and tasks, enhancing overall balance and stability.

11. Jumping Jacks

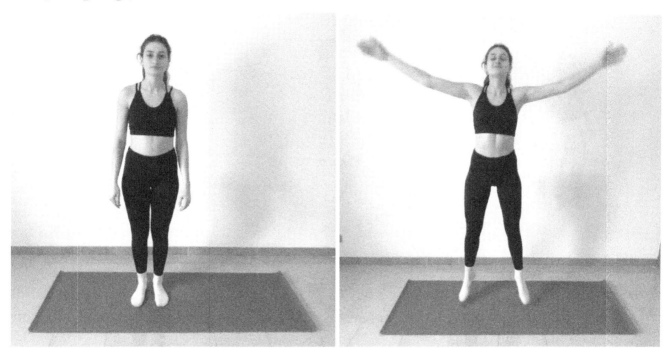

Setup:

1. Place a thick, sturdy mat on a flat surface.
2. Stand on the mat with your feet together and arms by your side.

How To Perform:

1. Begin to perform a jumping jack: jump up, spreading your legs wider than hip-width while simultaneously raising your arms above your head.
2. As you land, ensure your feet land softly on the mat, absorbing the impact through your knees.
3. Jump again, bringing your feet back together and your arms back to your sides. Repeat the movement with control and at a moderate pace.

Purpose:
This exercise promotes proprioceptive skills, enhancing the body's awareness of joint position, which is crucial for maintaining balance.
The dynamic nature of jumping jacks improves cardiovascular health, leg strength, and overall endurance, contributing to better balance and agility.

12. Rotational Jumps

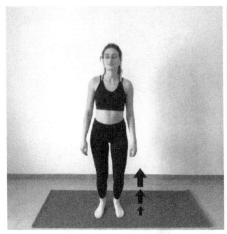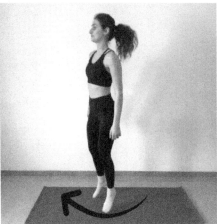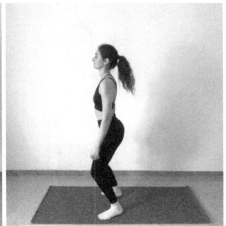

Setup:

1. Clear a safe space around you, ensuring there's enough room to jump and rotate without hitting anything.
2. Stand with your feet hip-width apart, knees slightly bent, ready to jump.

How To Perform:

1. Jump up and rotate your body 90 degrees to the left, landing softly with your knees bent to absorb the impact.
2. Immediately jump again, rotating back to the starting position. Ensure each landing is controlled and stable.
3. After completing a set rotating to the left, repeat the exercise by rotating to the right. Focus on smooth, controlled rotations and landings.

Purpose:

Rotational jumps improve dynamic balance and agility by challenging your body's ability to maintain stability through complex movements.

This exercise strengthens the core, legs, and glute muscles, all of which are essential for balance and powerful, controlled movements.

Enhancing rotational movement skills is crucial for daily activities and sports, offering better control over body movements and reducing the risk of falls during sudden changes in direction.

13. Yoga Warrior III Pose

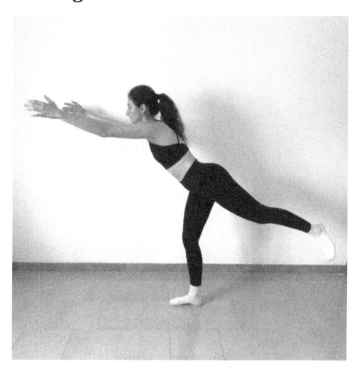

Setup:

1. Stand tall with your feet together, arms by your side.
2. Shift your weight to your right foot, preparing to lift your left leg.

How To Perform:

1. As you inhale, extend your arms forward, parallel to the ground.
2. Exhale, hinge at your hips, and lift your left leg behind you, simultaneously lowering your torso and arms forward until your body forms a T shape.
3. Keep your right leg strong, and your left leg, torso, and arms aligned and parallel to the floor. Gaze down to maintain neck alignment.
4. Hold the pose for several breaths, focusing on stability and balance. Slowly return to the starting position and repeat on the opposite side.

Purpose:
Warrior III pose challenges balance and stability by positioning the body in a dynamic alignment. This pose strengthens the ankles, legs, shoulders, and back while stretching the hamstrings and improving focus and concentration.

14. Pilates Swimming

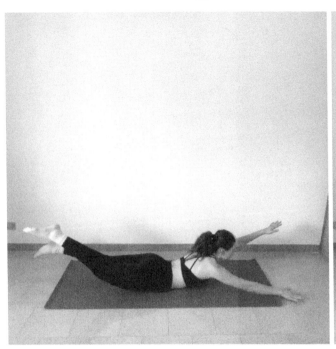 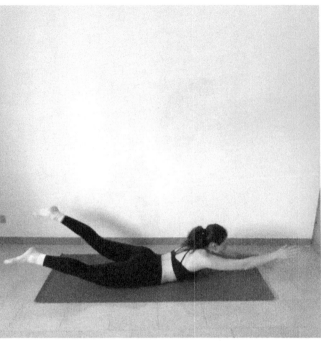

Setup:

1. Lie face down on a mat, with your arms extended in front of you and legs straight behind you.

How To Perform:

1. Lift your arms, legs, chest, and head off the mat, engaging your core and back muscles.
2. Begin to alternately lift your right arm and left leg higher, then switch to your left arm and right leg, mimicking a swimming motion.
3. Keep your gaze down to align your neck with your spine, and breathe steadily as you continue the alternating movements.
4. Perform the swimming motion for 30 seconds to 1 minute, maintaining a controlled and rhythmic pace.

Purpose:

Pilates swimming focuses on strengthening the back, core, and hip extensor muscles, all crucial for maintaining balance and posture.This exercise improves coordination and body awareness by challenging you to stabilize your core while moving your limbs independently.

4-Week Advanced Balance Challenge

This plan is crafted to challenge and improve your balance, flexibility, and overall body strength. Focused on advanced exercises, it aims to elevate your daily routine to new heights. Ensure to adapt the intensity according to your comfort and safety.

Week 1: Foundations of Strength

Day 1:

Exercise	Page	Sets & Repetitions / Duration
Lunges with Arm Lifts	p.58	3 sets x 10 reps
Yoga Tree Pose without Support	p.59	Hold for 30 seconds per side
Tai Chi Movements	p.65	5 minutes of continuous practice

Day 2:

Exercise	Page	Sets & Repetitions / Duration
Pilates Teaser	p.60	3 sets x 6 reps
Skater Hops	p.67	3 sets x 10 reps
Cone Taps	p.68	3 sets x 10 taps per side

Day 3:

Exercise	Page	Sets & Repetitions / Duration
Advanced Tandem Walk with Obstacles	p.61	3 rounds of a 10-foot walk
Jumping Jacks	p.69	3 sets x 15 reps
Rotational Jumps	p.70	2 sets x 10 reps

Day 4:

Exercise	Page	Sets & Repetitions / Duration
Single Leg Juggling	p.62	4 sets x 30 seconds juggling (Alternate legs after each set)
Cross-body Toe Touch	p.66	3 sets x 10 reps per side
Yoga Warrior III Pose	p.71	Hold for 20 seconds per side

Week 2: Elevating Stability

Day 1:

Exercise	Page	Sets & Repetitions / Duration
Pilates Swimming	p.72	Perform for 1 minute
Lunges with Arm Lifts	p.58	3 sets x 15 reps
Tai Chi Movements	p.65	5 minutes of continuous practice

Day 2:

Exercise	Page	Sets & Repetitions / Duration
Yoga Tree Pose without Support	p.59	Hold for 45 seconds per side
Skater Hops	p.67	3 sets x 12 reps
Jumping Jacks	p.69	3 sets x 20 reps

Day 3:

Exercise	Page	Sets & Repetitions / Duration
Advanced Tandem Walk with Obstacles	p.61	3 rounds of a 15-foot walk, increase obstacle difficulty
Cone Taps	p.68	3 sets x 12 taps per side
Pilates Teaser	p.60	3 sets x 8 reps

Day 4:

Exercise	Page	Sets & Repetitions / Duration
Rotational Jumps	p.70	3 sets x 12 reps
Single Leg Juggling	p.62	4 sets Increase juggling duration each set
Cross-body Toe Touch	p.66	Increase reach and speed, 3 sets x 12 reps per side

Week 3: Dynamic Harmony

Day 1:

Exercise	Page	Sets & Repetitions / Duration
Yoga Warrior III Pose	p.71	Hold for 30 seconds per side
Lunges with Arm Lifts	p.58	3 sets x 20 reps
Tai Chi Movements	p.65	6 minutes of continuous practice

Day 2:

Exercise	Page	Sets & Repetitions / Duration
Pilates Swimming	p.72	Perform for 2 minutes
Skater Hops	p.67	Increase distance of hops, 3 sets x 15 reps
Jumping Jacks	p.69	3 sets x 25 reps

Day 3:

Exercise	Page	Sets & Repetitions / Duration
Advanced Tandem Walk with Obstacles	p.61	Add dynamic movements, 3 rounds
Cone Taps	p.68	Include forward, lateral, and backward, 3 sets x 15 taps
Pilates Teaser	p.60	Add rotation, 3 sets x 10 reps

Day 4:

Exercise	Page	Sets & Repetitions / Duration
Rotational Jumps	p.70	4 sets x 15 reps
Single Leg Juggling	p.62	Juggle with alternate hands, 4 sets
Cross-body Toe Touch	p.66	Focus on fluid motion, 4 sets x 15 reps per side

Week 4: Mastery and Integration

Day 1:

Exercise	Page	Sets & Repetitions / Duration
Tai Chi Movements	p.65	7 minutes of continuous practice
Lunges with Arm Lifts	p.58	Incorporate dynamic arm movements, 3 sets x 20 reps
Pilates Swimming	p.72	Perform for 2 minutes

Day 2:

Exercise	Page	Sets & Repetitions / Duration
Yoga Tree Pose without Support	p.59	Incorporate arm movements, Hold for 1 minute per side
Skater Hops	p.67	Integrate arm swings, 3 sets x 20 reps
Advanced Tandem Walk with Obstacles	p.61	Use no visual aids, 3 rounds

Day 3:

Exercise	Page	Sets & Repetitions / Duration
Jumping Jacks	p.69	3 sets x 30 reps
Cone Taps	p.68	Blindfolded, 3 sets x 15 taps per side
Pilates Teaser	p.60	Perform with extended legs, 3 sets x 12 reps

Day 4:

Exercise	Page	Sets & Repetitions / Duration
Cross-body Toe Touch	p.66	Focus on fluid motion, 4 sets x 20 reps per side
Rotational Jumps	p.70	Increase rotation angle, 3 sets x 18 reps
Single Leg Juggling	p.62	Increase complexity, a ball in each hand, 3 sets

This plan is designed to progressively build your balance, coordination, and strength. It's essential to proceed with caution, especially with the more challenging exercises. Always ensure a safe environment to practice, and don't hesitate to modify any exercise to suit your level of comfort and capability.

Consistency and mindful practice are the keys to achieving balance mastery.

YOUR BONUS

I hope you're enjoying the book and that the exercises are helpful!

As promised, here is your bonus:

You just need to scan the QR code and you will have **EXCLUSIVE** access to our online platform, where you'll find all the videos of the exercises you've just seen.

This way, you can follow the workout routines without missing any exercise thanks to the support of the videos!

Happy reading,
Barbara

Vestibular System Workouts for Vertigo Management

Navigating through daily activities can become a daunting challenge for individuals experiencing vertigo. The vestibular system, an intricate part of our inner ear, plays a crucial role in maintaining balance and spatial orientation. When this system is disrupted, it can lead to feelings of dizziness, unsteadiness, and a spinning sensation, significantly impacting one's quality of life.

Understanding the importance of vestibular health, this section of the book is dedicated to vestibular system workouts specifically designed for vertigo management. These exercises are not just physical routines; they are a therapeutic journey towards regaining control over your balance and spatial awareness.

By gently challenging and stimulating the vestibular system, these workouts aim to desensitize you to the triggers of vertigo, improve your balance, and enhance your ability to perform daily tasks with confidence. Whether you're sitting at your desk, standing in line at the grocery store, or turning your head to converse with a friend, mastering these exercises will help you navigate your world with greater ease and stability.

Join us as we explore a series of targeted exercises, each carefully crafted to address the unique challenges faced by individuals managing vertigo. From simple head movements to more complex balance walks, these workouts are your stepping stones towards a more balanced and vertigo-free life.

1. Head Movements

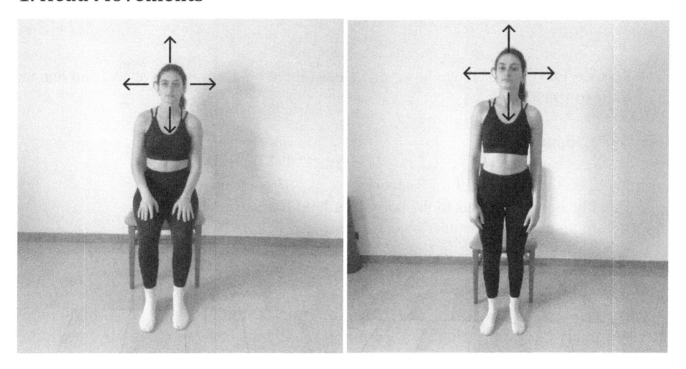

Setup:

1. Start by sitting in a sturdy chair without wheels.
2. Feet flat on the floor, hands on your thighs or by your sides.

How To Perform:

1. Slowly turn your head to the right as far as comfortable, hold for 3 seconds.
2. Return to the center and then turn your head to the left, hold for 3 seconds.
3. Gently tilt your head back to look up, then lower to look down, holding each for 3 seconds.
4. Stand up slowly, pause for a moment, and then repeat the head movements standing.
5. Perform 5 repetitions of each movement while sitting, then stand and repeat 5 more times.

Purpose:
This exercise aims to improve vestibular function by simulating everyday head movements. Transitioning from sitting to standing while performing these movements helps enhance balance and coordination, reducing dizziness and vertigo symptoms.

2. Gaze Stabilization

Setup:

1. Position two objects at eye level: one close (about an arm's length away) and one far (6 to 10 feet away).

How To Perform:

1. Focus on the near object for 3 seconds.
2. Quickly shift your focus to the far object, hold for 3 seconds.
3. Return your gaze to the near object.
4. Repeat the focus switch 10 times.

Purpose:
This exercise trains the eyes and brain to quickly and efficiently change focus between near and far objects, a common challenge for those with vestibular disorders. It aids in reducing vertigo triggered by rapid head or eye movements.

3. Balance Walk

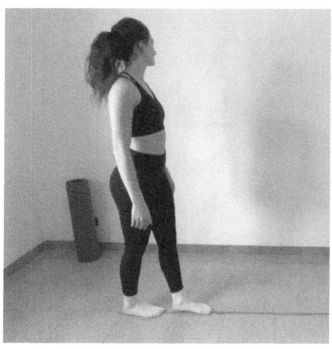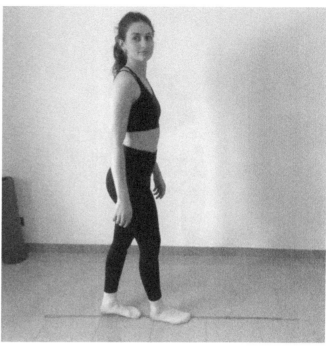

Setup:

1. Find a straight line on the floor or create one with tape.
2. Stand at one end of the line, feet together.

How To Perform:

1. Begin walking slowly along the line, placing one foot in front of the other, heel to toe.
2. As you walk, slowly turn your head left and right with each step.
3. Walk 10 steps forward, then carefully turn around and walk back.
4. Perform this walk 2-3 times.

Purpose:
This exercise enhances dynamic balance and vestibular stability by combining walking with controlled head movements. It's designed to simulate real-life situations where you must maintain balance while looking around.

4. Standing Sway

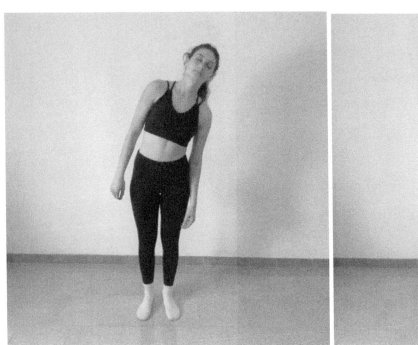 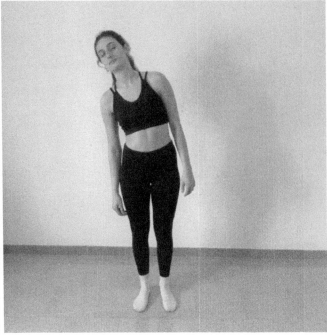

Setup:

1. Stand with your feet shoulder-width apart in a safe, open space.

How To Perform:

1. Begin with your eyes open, gently sway forward and backward, then side to side. Keep movements small and controlled.
2. Close your eyes and repeat the swaying motion, forward and back, then side to side.
3. Perform each sway direction for 30 seconds with eyes open, then 30 seconds with eyes closed.

Purpose:
Closing the eyes removes visual cues that help with balance, forcing the vestibular system and proprioception to work harder. This exercise strengthens the body's ability to maintain balance in both visually dependent and independent scenarios, crucial for managing vertigo.

Visual Coordination Exercises

In the journey to enhance balance and stability, visual coordination plays a pivotal role. The exercises you're about to explore are designed to refine the intricate dance between your eyes and brain, a fundamental aspect of maintaining equilibrium in both static and dynamic environments.

These activities are not just about seeing but about interpreting and reacting to visual information more effectively. Whether it's tracking a moving object without losing your balance or adjusting your posture in response to visual cues, the upcoming exercises will challenge and strengthen your visual coordination skills.

Perfect for individuals seeking to improve their balance through focused visual engagement, these exercises will guide you in developing sharper, more responsive visual coordination capabilities, essential for everyday activities and overall balance mastery.

Get ready to enhance your visual acuity and coordination, paving the way for a more stable and confident you.

1. Ball Toss and Catch

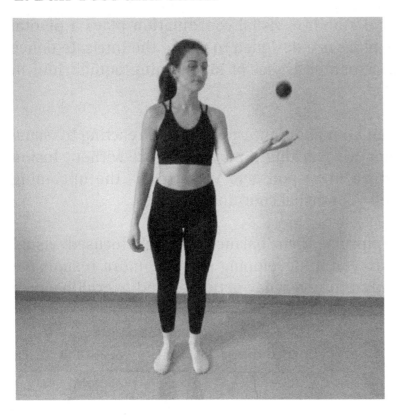

Setup:

1. Choose a soft ball that fits comfortably in your hand.
2. Stand or sit in a space where you have enough room to throw and catch the ball without obstructions.

How To Perform:

1. Start with the ball in your dominant hand.
2. Gently toss the ball upwards and catch it with the same hand. Repeat this 5 times.
3. Switch to your non-dominant hand and repeat the tossing and catching process 5 times.
4. For an added challenge, toss the ball from one hand and catch it with the other, alternating hands with each toss. Perform this for 10 repetitions (5 tosses per hand).

Purpose:
This exercise enhances hand-eye coordination and helps improve your focus and reaction times. It also trains your visual tracking skills, essential for maintaining balance during movement.

2. Tracking Moving Objects

Setup:

1. Attach a ball to a string or use a small pendulum.
2. Hang it from a height where you can comfortably see it without straining your neck.

How To Perform:

1. Stand or sit so that the ball is at eye level.
2. Gently push the ball to start it swinging.
3. Keep your head still, and follow the movement of the ball with your eyes only.
4. Track the ball for 30 seconds, then take a short break. Repeat this 3 times.

Purpose:

Improves your ability to track moving objects with your eyes, vital for activities that require precise visual coordination, such as walking in crowded spaces or catching.

3. Mirror Writing

Setup:

1. Place a mirror in front of you on a table.
2. Have a paper with letters or shapes you want to trace and a marker.

How To Perform:

1. Look into the mirror and use it to guide your hand as you trace the letters or shapes on the paper.
2. Try to complete the tracing without looking directly at your hand or the paper.
3. Perform this exercise for 5 minutes, focusing on accuracy and smoothness of your movements.

Purpose:

This exercise challenges your brain to adjust to mirrored visual feedback, enhancing cognitive processing and hand-eye coordination, which are crucial for maintaining balance and avoiding falls.

4. Dynamic Visual Acuity

Setup:

1. Have a partner move a book or tablet with text across your field of vision, or use a scrolling text app.
2. Sit or stand in a comfortable position.

How To Perform:

1. Focus on reading the text as it moves, trying to keep up with the pace without moving your head.
2. Start with slower movement and gradually increase the speed as you become more comfortable.
3. Continue this exercise for 5 minutes, taking breaks as needed.

Purpose:

Enhances your ability to focus on and interpret moving objects or information. This skill is essential for navigating dynamic environments safely, improving overall balance and spatial awareness.

Mind-Body Techniques for Enhanced Awareness

In the realm of balance and stability, the integration of mind and body practices offers a profound avenue for enhancing awareness and harmony.

The upcoming section, "Mind-Body Techniques for Enhanced Awareness," delves into exercises that transcend traditional physical training, inviting you to explore the serene interplay between mental focus, breath control, and precise movements.
These techniques are not just exercises; they are a journey towards inner peace, heightened awareness, and an increased sense of control over your body's movements and responses.

As you embark on this journey, you will discover practices rooted in ancient traditions, modernized for today's wellness enthusiasts. Each exercise is designed to fine-tune your attention, deepen your connection with your body, and cultivate a mindful presence that can significantly impact your balance and overall well-being.
Whether you're standing in a yoga pose, focusing on your breathing, or visualizing stability, these mind-body exercises serve as a bridge, enhancing your physical balance through mental clarity and emotional calmness.

Prepare to engage not just your muscles but your mind and spirit as well, as we explore exercises that will not only improve your physical balance but also bring about a greater sense of peace and presence in your daily life.

1. Tai Chi Basic Movements

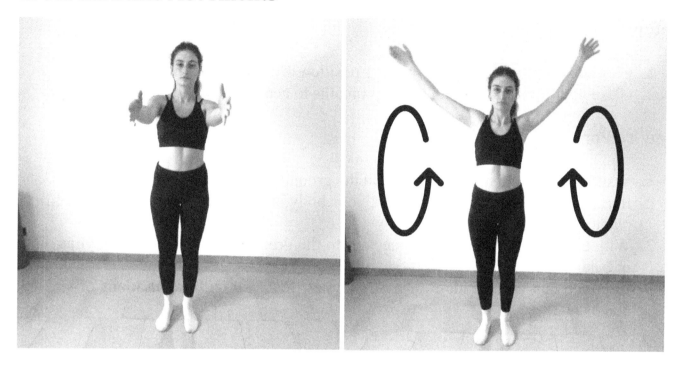

Setup:

1. Find a quiet, open space with enough room to move freely.
2. Stand with your feet shoulder-width apart, knees slightly bent.
3. Relax your shoulders and let your arms hang loosely by your sides.

How To Perform:

1. Begin with the "Wu Chi" stance: feet parallel, body relaxed, and mind focused.
2. Slowly raise your arms to chest height, palms down, as you inhale deeply.
3. As you exhale, gently lower your arms back to the starting position.
4. Perform the "Opening" move by separating your hands, moving them in a circular motion, and bringing them back together as if holding a ball.
5. Continue with 8-10 repetitions, focusing on the smooth flow of movements and synchronizing each movement with your breath.

Purpose:

Tai Chi movements are designed to improve balance and stability by enhancing body awareness, coordination, and promoting relaxation. The focus on breath helps to center the mind, reduce stress, and improve overall well-being.

2. Guided Imagery

Setup:

1. Choose a comfortable seated or lying position in a quiet environment.
2. Close your eyes and take a few deep breaths to center yourself.

How To Perform:

1. Visualize yourself standing firmly on the ground, feet rooted like a tree.
2. Imagine a gentle breeze that moves your body slightly, but your feet remain firmly planted.
3. With each breath, feel your connection to the ground deepen, enhancing your sense of balance and stability.
4. Continue this visualization for 5-10 minutes, focusing on the sensations of strength and balance.

Purpose:

Guided imagery enhances mental focus and concentration, which are crucial for maintaining balance. It helps in creating a mental model of stability, improving confidence in balance abilities.

3. Yoga Poses with Breath Work

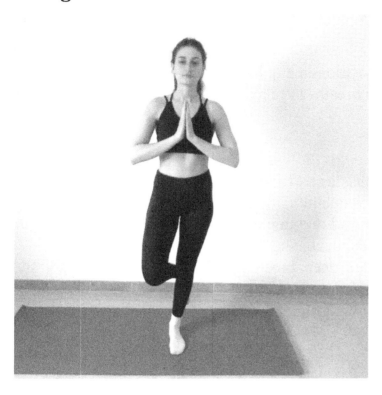

Setup:

1. Stand on a yoga mat or a non-slip surface for safety.
2. Begin in a standing position, feet hip-width apart, and hands at your sides.

How To Perform:

1. Shift your weight onto your left foot, and place the sole of your right foot on your left inner thigh or calf (avoid the knee).
2. Bring your palms together in front of your chest in a prayer position and focus on a point in front of you for balance.
3. Inhale deeply, and as you exhale, slowly raise your arms overhead, keeping your palms together.
4. Hold the pose for 5-10 breaths, then gently release and switch sides.

Purpose:
Yoga poses like the Tree Pose improve balance and stability by strengthening the legs and core. The integration of breath work aids in concentration, reduces stress, and enhances body awareness.

4. Progressive Muscle Relaxation

Setup:

1. Find a comfortable seated or lying position in a quiet, distraction-free area.
2. Close your eyes and take a few deep breaths to relax.

How To Perform:

1. Starting with your feet, tense the muscles as tightly as you can for 5 seconds, then release, focusing on the sensation of relaxation.
2. Move up through your body, tensing and relaxing each muscle group: calves, thighs, buttocks, abdomen, chest, arms, hands, neck, and face.
3. With each muscle group, incorporate deep breathing, inhaling as you tense, and exhaling as you release.
4. Continue until you've relaxed all muscle groups, focusing on the feeling of calmness and relaxation in your entire body.

Purpose:

Progressive muscle relaxation improves body awareness and reduces physical tension, which can negatively impact balance. It promotes relaxation, reduces stress, and can improve sleep quality, all of which contribute to better balance and stability.

Chapter 6: Lifestyle Adjustments for Better Balance

The Impact of Diet on Balance and Stability

The connection between diet and balance is often underestimated, yet nutrition plays a crucial role in maintaining and enhancing balance and stability as we age.
A well-balanced diet provides the vitamins, minerals, and energy our bodies need to sustain muscle strength, bone density, and overall physical function, which are essential components of good balance.

Nutrients such as calcium and vitamin D are vital for bone health, reducing the risk of osteoporosis, and maintaining a stable and strong posture. Meanwhile, proteins are essential for muscle maintenance and repair, supporting the muscular system that keeps us upright and balanced. Additionally, staying hydrated helps maintain the volume of blood circulating through the body, which is crucial for preventing dizziness and maintaining steady blood pressure levels.

A balanced diet that includes a variety of fruits, vegetables, lean proteins, whole grains, and healthy fats can provide these essential nutrients. Moreover, minimizing the intake of processed foods, which are often high in sugars and unhealthy fats, can help manage weight and reduce the risk of conditions that impair balance, such as diabetes and cardiovascular disease.

Suggested Weekly Meal Plan for Balance and Stability

Monday:
- **Breakfast**: Greek yogurt with mixed berries and a sprinkle of granola.
- **Lunch**: Grilled chicken salad with spinach, almonds, and avocados, dressed with olive oil and lemon.
- **Dinner**: Baked salmon with quinoa and steamed broccoli.

Tuesday:
- **Breakfast**: Oatmeal topped with sliced bananas and walnuts.
- **Lunch**: Turkey and hummus wrap with whole grain tortilla, cucumber, and tomato.
- **Dinner**: Stir-fried tofu with mixed vegetables and brown rice.

Wednesday:
- **Breakfast**: Smoothie with spinach, banana, almond milk, and a scoop of protein powder.

- **Lunch**: Lentil soup with a side of whole-grain bread.
- **Dinner**: Grilled lean steak with sweet potato and green beans.

Thursday:
- **Breakfast**: Scrambled eggs with mushrooms, onions, and a side of whole-wheat toast.
- **Lunch**: Quinoa salad with chickpeas, red bell pepper, and feta cheese.
- **Dinner**: Baked chicken breast with couscous and roasted asparagus.

Friday:
- **Breakfast**: Whole grain pancakes topped with fresh strawberries and a dollop of Greek yogurt.
- **Lunch**: Tuna salad with mixed greens, avocado, and cherry tomatoes.
- **Dinner**: Pasta with marinara sauce, grilled vegetables, and a side of lean ground turkey.

Saturday:
- **Breakfast**: Cottage cheese with pineapple chunks and a sprinkle of chia seeds.
- **Lunch**: Sushi rolls with miso soup and a seaweed salad.
- **Dinner**: Vegetable curry with lentils and brown rice.

Sunday:
- **Breakfast**: French toast made with whole-grain bread, topped with apple slices and cinnamon.
- **Lunch**: Grilled vegetable and goat cheese sandwich on whole-grain bread.
- **Dinner**: Roast chicken with roasted root vegetables and a side salad.

This meal plan incorporates a variety of nutrients that support balance and stability. Including at least three servings of dairy or fortified plant-based alternatives daily can ensure adequate intake of calcium and vitamin D. Including lean proteins at each meal supports muscle strength, and a variety of fruits and vegetables ensures a rich intake of vitamins and antioxidants.

Remember, hydration is key, so aim to drink at least 8 glasses of water throughout the day.

Modifying Your Environment to Prevent Falls

Creating a safe living environment is essential for preventing falls and maintaining balance as we age.

By making simple modifications in our homes, we can significantly reduce the risk of accidents, ensuring a safer and more comfortable space for daily activities.

Here are some practical tips for modifying your environment to prevent falls:

1. **Eliminate Tripping Hazards:** Scan your living space for potential tripping hazards such as loose rugs, electrical cords, and clutter. Secure rugs with non-slip pads or double-sided tape, organize cords away from walking paths, and keep floors clear of objects.

2. **Improve Lighting:** Ensure your home is well-lit to improve visibility, especially in hallways, staircases, and bathrooms. Consider installing brighter bulbs, night lights, and motion sensor lights that automatically illuminate dark areas as you approach.

3. **Install Handrails and Grab Bars:** Handrails on both sides of the stairways and grab bars in critical areas such as the shower, bathtub, and near the toilet can provide necessary support for maintaining balance and preventing slips.

4. **Non-Slip Surfaces:** Apply non-slip mats or decals in the bathtub and shower floor to prevent slipping on wet surfaces. Similarly, ensure that kitchen and bathroom floors are made of or covered with non-slip materials.

5. **Rearrange Furniture:** Arrange furniture to create clear, wide walking paths throughout your home. This organization helps avoid unnecessary obstacles that could contribute to falls.

6. **Adjust Height of Daily Use Items:** Keep everyday items within easy reach to avoid the need for stretching or bending that could lead to loss of balance. Use shelves and cabinets at waist or eye level for storage of frequently used objects.

7. **Wear Proper Footwear:** Inside the house, wear non-slip, supportive shoes instead of walking in socks or slippers with smooth soles. Proper footwear greatly reduces the risk of slipping.

8. **Stair Safety:** Ensure stairs are in good condition and consider adding contrasting color strips to the edge of each step to make them more visible. Also, keep staircases clutter-free.

9. **Emergency Access:** Keep a phone or emergency alert system accessible in case of a fall, ensuring you can call for help even if you're unable to get up.

By incorporating these modifications into your environment, you can create a safer living space that supports your balance and reduces the risk of falls. These changes, coupled with a balance-focused exercise routine, can help you maintain independence and improve your quality of life as you age.

Chapter 7: From Practice to Habit

Incorporating Balance Exercises into Daily Activities

Incorporating balance exercises into your daily routine is a crucial step towards enhancing your stability and reducing the risk of falls.

By making balance training a regular part of your life, you can seamlessly integrate these exercises into your daily activities, making it easier to maintain and improve your balance over time.

Here are strategies to help you incorporate balance exercises into your daily routine:

1. **Morning Routine Integration:** Start your day with simple balance exercises. While brushing your teeth or waiting for the coffee to brew, perform standing leg lifts or balance on one leg. This not only helps wake up your muscles but also sets a positive tone for the day.

2. **Work or Desk Breaks:** If you spend a lot of time sitting at a desk, use short breaks to practice balance exercises. Stand up, stretch, and try a few balance poses like the tandem stand or heel-to-toe walk. These breaks can help reduce stiffness and improve circulation, besides boosting your balance.

3. **While Watching TV:** Utilize commercial breaks or the end of episodes as cues to stand up and engage in a few minutes of balance training. Practice exercises such as standing marches, side leg raises, or even gentle yoga poses focused on balance.

4. **Incorporate into Chores:** Turn mundane chores into opportunities for balance training. For instance, while washing dishes, practice shifting your weight from one foot to the other. When vacuuming or sweeping, use the moment to strengthen your stance and engage your core.

5. **Outdoor Activities:** Engage in outdoor activities that naturally improve balance, such as walking on uneven surfaces, gardening, or gentle hiking. These activities not only offer a change of scenery but also challenge your balance in varied and practical ways.

6. **Socialize with Movement:** Whenever possible, choose social activities that involve movement and balance. Joining a dance class, walking group, or tai chi practice with friends can make balance exercises more enjoyable and motivating.

7. **Mindful Movement:** Incorporate mindfulness into your balance exercises by paying close attention to your body's movements and sensations. This practice enhances the connection between your mind and body, improving your balance and coordination.

8. **Evening Wind Down:** End your day with a few calming balance exercises as part of your evening routine. Gentle yoga poses or tai chi movements can help relax your body and mind, preparing you for a restful night's sleep.

By embedding balance exercises into your daily activities, you transform them from isolated tasks into natural parts of your lifestyle.

This approach not only helps improve your balance but also ensures that you consistently work on maintaining it, leading to long-term benefits for your health and well-being.

Tracking Your Progress: Tools and Tips

Tracking your progress is an essential component of any balance exercise program. By monitoring your improvements over time, you can stay motivated, adjust your routine as needed, and celebrate your successes.

Here are some tools and tips to effectively track your balance exercise progress:

1. **Exercise Journal:** Keep a dedicated exercise journal to record your daily balance activities. Note the exercises you perform, the number of repetitions, and any changes in difficulty or assistance needed. Over time, this journal will provide a clear picture of your progress and areas for improvement.

2. **Balance Test Recordings:** Regularly perform self-assessment balance tests (as outlined in earlier chapters) and record your results. Comparing these results over weeks or months can help you see tangible improvements in your balance capabilities.

3. **Video Diaries:** Consider recording yourself performing balance exercises periodically. Watching these videos can help you visually assess your progress, form, and posture improvements. It's also a motivational tool to see how far you've come.

4. **Apps and Wearables:** Utilize fitness apps and wearable devices that track physical activity. Some apps and devices have features specifically designed to monitor balance and stability exercises, offering insights into your performance and progress.

5. **Goal Setting:** Set specific, measurable, achievable, relevant, and time-bound (SMART) goals for your balance training. Review and adjust these goals regularly based on your tracking journal and test results. Celebrating when you reach these goals can be a powerful motivator.

6. **Feedback from Professionals:** If possible, work with a physical therapist or fitness trainer who can provide professional assessments of your balance. Their expert feedback can help fine-tune your exercise program and offer objective insights into your progress.

7. **Buddy System:** Partner with a friend or family member who is also working on improving their balance. Share your progress, challenges, and successes. This social support can boost motivation and provide an external perspective on your improvements.

8. **Reflective Practice:** Regularly take time to reflect on how improvements in balance affect your daily life. Note any activities that have become easier or any reductions in stumbles or falls. This qualitative assessment can be just as rewarding as quantitative measurements.

By employing a combination of these tracking tools and tips, you can gain a comprehensive understanding of your balance exercise journey.

This not only helps in maintaining motivation but also ensures that your exercise regimen continues to meet your evolving needs, leading to sustained improvements in balance and overall health.

Chapter 8: Navigating Life's Balance Challenges

Emergency Preparedness: What to Do After a Fall

Falling can be a frightening and dangerous experience, especially for seniors. Being prepared and knowing how to respond after a fall is crucial to minimizing injuries and complications.

This section will guide you through steps to take immediately after a fall and how to prepare for such events in the future.

1. **Stay Calm:** The first step after a fall is to remain calm. Take deep breaths and assess your situation without making any sudden movements.

2. **Assess for Injuries:** Carefully evaluate yourself for any injuries. If you are hurt, try to avoid moving and call for help using a phone, medical alert system, or by shouting for someone nearby.

3. **Getting Up Safely:** If you feel strong enough to get up, do so slowly. Roll onto your side, push yourself up to a sitting position, and pause for a moment. Find a sturdy piece of furniture, such as a chair, to pull yourself up. Take your time, and once standing, pause again to ensure you are steady before moving.

4. **Seek Medical Attention:** Even if you feel fine, it's important to consult a healthcare professional after a fall to check for any injuries that might not be immediately apparent, such as concussions or fractures.

5. **Review the Cause:** Analyze what caused the fall. Was it a trip hazard, balance issue, or something else? Identifying the cause can help you make necessary changes to prevent future falls.

6. **Emergency Plan:** Have an emergency plan in place. This includes keeping a phone or medical alert device within reach at all times, maintaining a list of emergency contacts in an accessible location, and informing family or friends about your plan.

7. **Exercise and Strength Training:** Incorporate balance and strength exercises into your routine to improve your stability and reduce the risk of future falls. Practices such as Tai Chi, yoga, and Pilates can be particularly beneficial.

8. **Home Safety Check:** Regularly perform a home safety check to identify and mitigate potential fall hazards, such as loose rugs, cluttered walkways, and poor lighting.

9. **Wear Appropriate Footwear:** Always wear shoes that provide good support and have non-slip soles, both indoors and outdoors.

By taking these steps, you can significantly reduce your risk of falling and ensure that you are prepared to handle such situations should they arise.
Remember, prevention and preparedness are key to maintaining your independence and well-being.

Complementary Practices: Chair Yoga, Tai Chi, and Pilates

Incorporating complementary practices such as chair yoga, Tai Chi, and Pilates into your routine can significantly enhance balance, flexibility, and overall well-being.

These gentle yet effective exercises are particularly beneficial for seniors seeking to improve their stability and reduce the risk of falls.
Here, we explore how each practice contributes to better balance and how you can integrate them into your daily life.

Chair Yoga

Chair yoga offers a safe and accessible way to enjoy the benefits of yoga, especially for individuals with mobility issues or those who find standing exercises challenging. This practice involves seated poses and stretches that improve flexibility, muscle strength, and joint health. Chair yoga also focuses on deep breathing and mindfulness, promoting relaxation and stress reduction.

- **How to Start:** Begin with simple seated poses, focusing on gentle stretches and mindful breathing. Classes are often available at community centers or online.

For those interested in exploring Chair Yoga further, we've also written a comprehensive book titled:

"Chair Yoga for Seniors Over 60: How to Reclaim Independence, Mobility, Balance and Lose Weight in Only 10 Minutes a Day with A Simple 28-Day Challenge (50+ Illustrated Exercises)."

This guide is specifically designed to cater to the needs of seniors, providing you with the tools to enhance your independence, mobility, and balance through chair yoga. Whether you're new to yoga or looking to adapt your practice to suit your current abilities, this book offers a practical and impactful way to incorporate yoga into your daily life.

Tai Chi

Tai Chi is a Chinese martial art known for its slow, graceful movements and deep breathing techniques. Practicing Tai Chi improves balance by enhancing proprioception (the sense of body position) and strengthening the muscles used for stability. It's also effective in reducing stress and improving mental focus.

- **How to Start:** Look for Tai Chi classes designed for beginners or seniors. Many community centers and gyms offer classes, and there are also instructional videos available online.

Pilates

Pilates focuses on core strength, flexibility, and mindful movement, making it an excellent choice for improving balance and stability. While traditional Pilates involves floor exercises, many adaptations are suitable for seniors, including the use of equipment like reformers and chairs to assist with movements.

- **How to Start:** Start with beginner classes that focus on core strengthening and stability exercises. Pilates classes specifically designed for seniors can provide a supportive and accessible environment to learn.

-

Integrating into Your Routine

- **Schedule Regular Sessions:** Dedicate specific times each week to practice these exercises, ensuring consistency in your routine.

- **Combine Practices:** Consider combining elements of chair yoga, Tai Chi, and Pilates into your weekly exercise routine to enjoy a variety of benefits.

- **Attend Guided Classes:** Participating in classes led by qualified instructors can provide you with personalized guidance and support.

- **Practice Mindfulness:** In addition to physical exercises, incorporate mindfulness and breathing exercises into your daily routine to enhance mental well-being.

By embracing these complementary practices, you can enjoy a holistic approach to improving balance and stability, reducing the risk of falls, and enhancing your overall quality of life.

Whether you're practicing chair yoga for flexibility, Tai Chi for balance, or Pilates for core strength, each activity offers unique benefits that contribute to a healthier, more balanced lifestyle.

Conclusion

The Journey Ahead: Maintaining Balance for Life

As we conclude this comprehensive guide on balance exercises, it's important to reflect on the journey you've embarked upon and the strides you've made towards achieving and maintaining balance in your life.

Embracing the exercises and techniques outlined in this book is not just about preventing falls or enhancing physical stability; it's about enriching your quality of life, fostering independence, and empowering yourself to live fully and confidently at any age.

Balance is more than a physical attribute; it's a cornerstone of a vibrant, active lifestyle.
By dedicating time to the exercises and practices we've discussed, you're not only improving your physical well-being but also investing in your mental and emotional health. The discipline and mindfulness you cultivate through balance training can have profound effects on all aspects of your life, from how you navigate physical challenges to how you manage stress and embrace the present moment.

As you move forward, remember that maintaining balance is an ongoing journey. There will be days when you feel strong and centered, and others when maintaining balance might seem more challenging. These fluctuations are a natural part of life. What's important is your commitment to persist, adapt, and approach each day with a positive and proactive mindset.

Celebrate the progress you've made, no matter how small it may seem. Every step taken is a step towards greater stability, confidence, and independence. Encourage yourself to explore new activities, perhaps integrating complementary practices like Chair yoga, Tai Chi, or Pilates into your routine to further enhance your balance and overall well-being.

Finally, let this book serve not only as a guide but as a companion on your journey to balance mastery.
Revisit it whenever you need a refresher, share it with friends who might benefit from its teachings, and continue to seek out new ways to challenge and improve your balance.

The path to maintaining balance for life is both rewarding and enriching, and it's a journey well worth pursuing.

Congratulations on taking this significant step towards a balanced and fulfilling life. Here's to your health, happiness, and stability, today and in the years to come.

Your Opinion is Fundamental

As we close this chapter of your balance journey, we hope this guide has been a valuable resource in guiding you towards a more stable and confident life. Your progress and commitment to improving your balance are truly commendable, and we believe your experiences can inspire and encourage others who are embarking on similar paths.

If this book has made a positive impact on your journey towards better balance, we kindly ask you to share your thoughts and experiences by leaving a review. Your feedback is not only fundamental to us but can also be a beacon of hope and a source of motivation for others looking to improve their balance and overall well-being.

Thank you for allowing us to be a part of your journey to improved balance and for considering leaving a review. Together, we can inspire a movement towards healthier, more balanced living for seniors everywhere.